Geriatric Medicine

Geriatric Medicine

NICHOLAS CONI
MA FRCP FRCP(C)
Consultant Emeritus

CLAIRE NICHOLL
MB FRCP
Consultant Physician & Associate Lecturer

STEPHEN WEBSTER
MD FRCP
Consultant Emeritus

K. JANE WILSON
MB MRCP
Consultant Physician & Associate Lecturer

All of
Department of Medicine for the Elderly
Addenbrooke's Hospital, Cambridge

Sixth edition

Blackwell
Publishing

First published 1977   Reprinted 1989   Fifth edition 1998
Second edition 1980   Fourth edition 1993   Reprinted 1999, 2000
Reprinted 1984, 1986   Reprinted 1993, 1996   Sixth edition 2003
Third edition 1988

Library of Congress Cataloging-in-Publication Data

Lecture notes on geriatric medicine / Nicholas Coni . . . [et al.].–6th ed.
    p.;   cm. — (Lecture notes)
Rev. ed. of: Lecture notes on geriatrics/Nicholas Coni, Stephen Webster. 5th ed. 1998.
Includes bibliographical references and index.
    ISBN 1-4051-0162-8
    1. Geriatrics — Outlines, syllabi, etc.
    [DNLM: 1. Geriatrics. WT 100 L471 2003]
    I. Coni, Nicholas. II. Coni, Nicholas. Lecture notes on geriatrics. III. Series: Lecture notes series
    (Blackwell Scientific Publications)
RC952 .C583 2003
618.97 — dc21   2002153105

ISBN 1-4051-0162-8

A catalogue record for this title is available from the British Library

Set in 9/11 ^{1}/$_2$ pt Gill Sans by SNP Best-set Typesetter Ltd., Hong Kong
Printed and bound in India by Replika Press Pvt. Ltd.

Commissioning Editor: Vicki Noyes
Production Editor: Jonathan Rowley
Production Controller: Chris Downs

For further information on Blackwell Publishing, visit our website:
http://www.blackwellpublishing.com

Contents

Preface to the Sixth Edition

Those readers familiar with previous editions will note two obvious changes as soon as they see the cover of this, the sixth edition. The first is the title. *Geriatrics*, as a substantive, started to become debased many years ago when certain sections of the media began bestowing this title on persons of advanced years, especially if they showed the slightest evidence of cognitive decline or even mild memory impairment. It thus acquired a pejorative connotation, and many hospital departments therefore took refuge in the bland title of 'medicine for the elderly'. But the word makes an etymologically respectable adjective, even if not a particularly euphonious one, and describes the medical specialty in terms immediately understood throughout the profession.

The second change is far more important, and that is the addition of two new authors. Old geriatricians *do* die, *and* they *do* fade away, and it is essential for any medical text to be regularly brought up to date. The 2001 census showed for the first time a preponderance of people aged over 60 over those aged under 16 and so geriatric medicine is increasingly becoming *normal* medicine. The rapid changes in every branch of medicine thus affect geriatric medicine as profoundly as any other field — indeed, more so than most, as old people belatedly assert their status as legitimate subjects of medical endeavour. It is therefore necessary for authors to be abreast of the 'cutting edge' of the advances being made almost daily in *geriatric medicine*.

There is endless fascination in trying to help patients of advanced age, and great satisfaction to be gained when, often to their surprise, one succeeds in doing so. Older people often have life histories and personalities of great richness, but unravelling the histories of their illnesses can be a major challenge. A vague complaint of slowing down, or becoming a little unsteady, or loss of appetite, can indicate one of so many possible underlying diseases. Identifying the various pathologies, some new, some old, that they may have acquired *en route* through life, together with the pills accumulated in various attempts to treat them all, and then to tease out which of these illnesses may be responsible for the recent decline in quality of life: which are readily susceptible to treatment and which are not: how burdensome the treatment might be in view of the general state of health and probable life expectancy and whether to comply with the patient's expressed view that it is all a waste of effort at his or her age, or to dismiss that view as due to natural despondency which might be totally reversed if well-being could be restored — all this requires a modicum of time and, we suggest, of wisdom. In younger age groups, a single diagnosis is usually sufficient to explain the symptoms, and then the treatment can be readily looked up in any reference book. Dealing with the aged requires the deployment of the *art* of medicine, and the complexities of these issues and the publicity surrounding some of them have necessitated a new chapter on the legal and ethical aspects of geriatric practice.

NKC
CGN
SGPW
KJW
Cambridge
October 2002

Abbreviations

A & E	accident and emergency
ABGs	arterial blood gases
ACA	anterior cerebral artery
ACE	angiotensin-converting enzyme
AD	Alzheimer's disease
ADH	antidiuretic hormone
ADL	activities of daily living
AF	atrial fibrillation
AFB	acid-fast bacillus
AIDS	acquired immune deficiency syndrome
AMT	Abbreviated Mental Test
ANS	autonomic nervous system
AP	anterior pituitary
AV	atrioventricular
AVP	arginine vasopressin
BCC	basal cell carcinoma
BMD	bone mineral density
BMI	body mass index
BNF	British National Formulary
BP	blood pressure
CABG	coronary artery bypass graft
CAPD	continuous ambulatory peritoneal dialysis
CCF	congestive cardiac failure
CHI	Commission for Health Improvement
CK	creatine kinase
CK-MB	isoenzyme of creatine kinase with muscle and brain subunits
CNS	central nervous system
CO	carbon monoxide
CO_2	carbon dioxide
COHb	carboxyhaemoglobin
COPD	chronic obstructive pulmonary disease
CPNs	Community Psychiatric Nurses
CPR	cardiopulmonary resuscitation
CRP	C-reactive protein
CSF	cerebrospinal fluid
CSM	carotid sinus massage
CT	computerized tomography
CVA	cerebrovascular accident
CVP	central venous pressure
CXR	chest X-ray

DC	direct-current
DIC	disseminated intravascular coagulation
DIPs	distal interphalangeals
DMARDS	disease modifying anti-rheumatic drugs
DVT	deep venous thrombosis
DEXA	dual energy X-ray absorptiometry
ECG	electrocardiogram
ECT	electroconvulsive therapy
EEG	electroencephalogram/graphy
EMG	electromyography/electromyogram
EOFAD	early-onset familial Alzheimer's disease
ESR	erythrocyte sedimentation rate
FBC	full blood count
FEV_1	forced expiratory volume in 1 second
FSH	follicle-stimulating hormone
FVC	forced vital capacity
GDS	Geriatric Depression Score
GI	gastrointestinal
GP	general practitioner
HImPs	Health Improvement Plans
HIV	human immunodeficiency virus
I^{131}	iodine-131
ICA	internal carotid artery
IgG	immunoglobulin G
IHD	ischaemic heart disease
i.m.	intramuscularly
INR	international normalized ratio
ITU	intensive care/therapy unit
i.v.	intravenous
LacI	lacunar infarct
LDH	lactate dehydrogenase
LDL-C	low density lipoprotein cholestrol
LH	luteinizing hormone
LMN	lower-motor neuron
LMWH	low molecular weight heparin
LOAD	late-onset Alzheimer's disease
LOC	loss of consciousness
LTOT	long-term oxygen therapy
LV	left ventricular
LVH	left ventricular hypertrophy
MCA	middle cerebral artery
MGUS	monoclonal gammopathy of unknown significance
MI	myocardial infarction/infarct
MMSE	Mini-Mental State Examination
MNA	Mini-Nutritional Assessment
MRI	magnetic resonance imaging
MRSA	methicillin-resistant *Staphylococcus aureus*
MS	multiple sclerosis
MSU	mid-stream urine

NBM	nil by month
NCSE	non-convulsive status epilepticus
NG	nasogastric
NHS	National Health Service
NICE	National Institute for Clinical Excellence
NMDA	N-methyl-D-aspartate
NOF	neck of femur
NSAIDs	non-steroidal anti-inflammatory drugs
OTC	over the counter
PA	pernicious anaemia
PACI	partial anterior circulatory infarct
PD	Parkinson's disease
PE	pulmonary embolism
PEG	percutaneous endoscopic gastrostomy
PIPs	proximal interphalangeals
POCI	posterior circulatory infarct
PPARγ	peroxisome proliferator activated receptor gamma
PSA	prostate specific antigen
PTCA	percutaneous transluminal coronary angioplasty
RA	right atrium
RAS	renal artery stenosis
rt-PA	recombinant tissue-type plasminogen activator
SAH	subarachnoid haemorrhage
SCC	squamous cell carcinoma
SDH	subdural haematoma
SE	status epilepticus
SERMS	selective oestrogen modulators
Sesta MIBI scan	technitium 99m methoxy isobutyl isonitrile
SIADH	syndrome of inappropriate antidiuretic hormone
SLE	systemic lupus erythematosus
SN	substantia nigra
SOL	space-occupying lesion
SSRIs	selective serotonin reuptake inhibitors
T_3	triiodothyronine
T_4	thyroxine
TACI	total anterior circulatory infarct
TB	tuberculosis
TEDS	thromboembolic device stockings
TFTs	thyroid-function tests
TIA	transient ischaemic attack
TOE	transoesophageal echocardiography
tPA	tissue plasminogen activator
TSH	thyroid-stimulating hormone
TURP	transurethral prostatectomy
U & Es	urea and electrolytes
UKPDS	United Kingdom Prospective Diabetes Study
UMN	upper motor neuron
V/Q	ventilation/perfusion
WBC	white blood cells

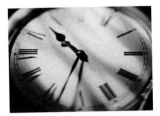

The World Grows Old

Introduction

If the 20th century was the period when the Western World turned grey, it is to be hoped that the 21st century will be the time when it wakes up to the new situation and begins to make appropriate plans for services. There is some evidence that this is occurring. The increasing presence of elderly people is now recognized in plays, films, soap operas and comedy series.

The common afflictions of old age are now well recognized, not as a cause for shame and disgrace, but as serious diseases. Examples are the public information about the dementia of ex-President Reagan of the USA and a dramatization of the same disease as it affected the famous philosopher and novelist Iris Murdoch. Middle-aged, middle class articulate 'children' such as Michael Ignatief, Linda Grant and Margaret Mason have written in detail about the dementing process as it affected their parents, themselves and their families. John Mortimer has described the problems associated with visual impairment in his elderly father and he now writes amusingly about his own infirmities of old age.

The Human Rights Act 1998 (adopted by the UK on 2nd October 2000) has the potential to offer protection to vulnerable elderly people, especially Articles 2, 3, 8, 10 and 14 (see box). This Act applies to all public bodies, i.e. the NHS and Local Authority Social Service Departments.

Human Rights Act 1998

Article 2	Right to life
Article 3	Prohibition of torture and inhuman and degrading treatment
Article 8	Right to respect for private and family life and home
Article 10	Freedom of expression and right to information
Article 14	Right not to be discriminated against

Population trends (Table 1.1)

There are marked differences between the developed and developing countries, e.g. France took 115 years (1865–1980) to double the proportion of elderly people (7–14%) whereas China's proportion will double between 2000 and 2027. The prime reason for the worldwide increase in the proportion of elderly subjects is the combined effect of declining child mortality and a falling birth rate. Consequences and solutions will depend on the levels of economic and educational development within individual countries. By 2030 most countries will have a similar age structure.

Developed countries

• There has been a dramatic rise in the elderly throughout the past 100 years but this is now slowing down (Fig. 1.1).

1

PREDICTED ELDERLY POPULATIONS IN 2025	
China	198 343
India	107 713
Indonesia	24 816
Brazil	21 945
Mexico	12 829
UK	12 912
Nigeria	9115

Table 1.1 Predicted elderly population (over 65 years in thousands) in 2025.

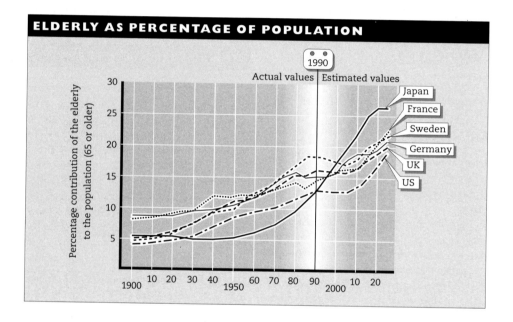

Fig. 1.1 Percentage contribution of the elderly to the overall population in advanced Western countries and Japan.

• However, the old old, i.e. greater than 75 years of age, are still increasing rapidly. In the UK the over-85s will continue to double every 30 years (1961, 300 000; 1991, 800 000; 2021, 1 500 000).
• A sophisticated medical service is established.
• Specialist services are available for the elderly.
• The rising expectations of the elderly, their supports and carers will result in rising costs.
• Population trends in the UK alone demand a 1% increase in health funding in addition to inflation and costs due to technological development.
• Ethical dilemmas will be more pressing, e.g. prolongation of death by technological intervention or medicated survival of young chronic sick and acutely ill frail elderly patients.
• Financial consequences of decisions must be calculated and proper provisions made to support the choice made. An elderly person costs the health services nine times as much as a young person.
• A century ago, i.e. 1900, more children under 1 year of age died each year than people under the age of 65 now die each year—see Table 1.2 showing changes in the death rate over time.

UK MORTALITY RATES FOR YOUNG AND OLD	
1919 UK	12% of deaths in 1st year of life 65% of deaths before age 65 years
2002 UK	<1% of deaths in 1st year of life. 19% of deaths before age 65 years

Table 1.2 Death, formerly common in infancy and usual before 65 years, is now rare in infancy and unusual before 65 years.

• By 2015 in the UK it is predicted that the over 65s will begin to outnumber those under 16 years of age.

• The Commission on Global Ageing warns of the risk of 'ageing recessions' due to a fall in the size of workforce numbers (labour shortages) plus increased service demands (caring services). The peak risk is in 2010, but Japan has already been affected.

• Increasing anxiety concerning future poverty in old age, due to shrinkage in state benefits, reluctance of 'the young' to invest in pension schemes and the unreliability of financial services in regard to pension provision.

• Medical training continues to concentrate on increasing super/sub-specialization, thus leading to practitioners unable to cope with complex aetiologies (sociological, psychological and medical) and multi-pathology (co-morbidity) and the atypical presentations which are common in elderly patients, i.e. a mis-match between aspirations of young medics and their elderly patients.

• Community care is quite rightly individually based and very varied. Comparisons between countries is therefore very difficult due to variations in taxation policy, population density and political climate. It is, however, easier to make comparisons with regards to institutional care, usually in residential or nursing homes. Even here there are wide variations from the UK with 4% of persons over 65 years of age in care homes to the USA at almost 6% and the Netherlands at almost 11%.

• The historical development of the patterns of care are similar. In all societies, there has always been a heavy reliance on self-sufficiency and family care. In these circumstances, the healthy old and the wealthy old have always faired the best. For the more disadvantaged, there has always been a need to rely on support from non-family members.

• In the 'Old World', this non-family support was originally provided by the church or by occupationally related charities or guilds. In England, the state began to become more prominent in the 17th century with the first Poor Law Act, which provided workhouse care and 'outdoor relief' (through community support, usually financial). This continued until the end of the 19th century. The 20th century saw the beginning of the welfare state—gradually growing in the first half of the century and reaching a peak at mid-century and then declining towards the end of the 1980s. At the time of decline, the general move was away from the provision of services by the state to the regulation of provision of services supplied by other organizations. This regulation has gradually been devolved and often diluted with the central control gradually lost or weakened. This trend has been most marked in the USA, but is now apparent in Australasia and the UK.

• In the USA, 67% of nursing homes are run by profit making organizations (increasingly large multi-national companies). In 1999, one of the largest companies also had large numbers of beds in Europe and Australia. However, the for-profit companies have a worse record for staffing levels (20% less than non-profit making institutions) and skill mix, and a higher incidence of violations of standards. The regulatory arrangements are clearly failing to improve or even maintain standards. Public control appears

to have been lost and for every dollar spent in the for-profit area, less than 26 cents is spent on care.
• In Australia, the proportion of for-profit nursing home beds was historically about 27%, but had risen to 55% by the year 2000. Between 1996 and 2000, the cost of public funding of private nursing homes rose from $A2.5 billion to $A3.9 billion. The cost of the regulatory system has doubled, but it appears to be weakening as unannounced inspections ceased, reports of inspections became more difficult to obtain and available sanctions were rarely used.

Developing countries

• Currently they have 50% of the world's elderly population — will rise to 75% by the year 2020.
• These countries are about to experience a massive and rapid distortion of previous population patterns, the rate of increase in the elderly population will be up to 15 times that of the UK (e.g. in Colombia, the Philippines and Thailand).
• Rising number of elderly people will coincide with falling birth rate, as contraceptive policies become effective.
• Their health services are often primitive, patchy and inappropriate to needs.
• There are many other pressing financial demands for expansion, e.g. education, housing and development of infrastructure.
• Economic dependence on developed countries is restrictive.
• Political instability is common.

• Social structure likely to be rapidly altered, e.g. by population migration and reduced infant mortality.
• Potentially preventable disabilities acquired in youth will complicate old age.
• The poor will be unable to acquire sufficient wealth to provide for themselves in old age; therefore the total burden will either fall on the state or will be neglected.
• European studies show that the survival of babies with low birth-weight and reduced growth in the 1st year leads to poor adult health — especially regarding BP and blood sugar control. This is likely to have significant consequences in India and southeast Asia in the future.
• Globalization via the World Trade Organization will attempt to maintain high drug costs and introduce insurance schemes that will cherry-pick the affluent/well and leave the disadvantaged to the struggling public services. There is also likely to be encouragement of inappropriate 'high-tech' procedures. World trade also tends to encourage development of bad health habits; e.g. smoking tobacco, excess use of alcohol and the recreational use of drugs.
• Population patterns at risk of distortion by epidemics, e.g. HIV/AIDS.
• It is a false assumption that elderly people in undeveloped countries are not a problem because they are so few. They do exist and their life expectancy at 65 years is very similar in both developed and undeveloped countries — see Table 1.3.
• Doctors and nurses training in the undeveloped countries need expertise in elderly care because of the changing demography of their own countries and the tendency for them to be 'poached' by developed countries where they

LIFE EXPECTANCY AT 65 YEARS

	Developed countries (Years)	Undeveloped countries (Years)
Women	19	15
Men	16	12

Table 1.3.

may find themselves confronted by very elderly patients for the first time.

Ageing in India

The descriptions of facilities for 'care' in this book (as opposed to 'cure') of elderly people will be representative of the Western World, especially of the UK. This is because national variation is great and space is limited. With regards to the less developed countries, information is often very limited and sometimes unreliable. These restrictions apply to information about India, but at least statistics are being collected. To illustrate some of the differences between the East and the West, we have included information from the WHO publication *Ageing in India*, published in 1999. Life expectancy at the age of 60 in India has increased for both men and women between 1961 and 2001 by 3–4 years, and is now 15.2 years for men and 16.4 years for women. Table 1.4 shows commonest diseases and disabilities in the elderly population in India. It should be noted that, as is the case worldwide, cardiovascular disease takes pole position. Some 60–75% of elderly people in India are economically dependent, usually on their family. However, the extended family is disappearing and the social status of elderly people is being eroded. Since 1992, an old age pension has been available for those with no means of support at a level of approximately US $1.00 per month. Services for elderly people are very few and far between. In 1997, there was reported to be only 354 old people homes, usually organized by charities.

Population of UK			
	1971	1996	2061
<16 years old	25%	21%	17%
>65 years old	13%	16%	24%
In 2015 population <16 years = >65 years			

Population of India	
Year 2000	7% over 60 years of age
Year 2025	12% over 60 years of age

Ageing in Africa

Ageing in Africa is different to other areas. It provides an example of how the unexpected can undermine projections. The effects of AIDS and war are seriously distorting the age patterns of this continent.

United Nations reports indicate that half of teenagers in Africa will die from AIDS. In Botswana about two-thirds of 15 year olds will die before reaching the age of 50. Many African children have been orphaned by AIDS, and their grandmothers have taken over the parenting role as the 'middle generation' has been decimated by early death. These early deaths will seriously distort the age of the available workforce in Africa.

A World Health Organization Report 2001 calculated that the annual worldwide rate of war casualties is about one-third of a million, that over half of these (54%) will occur in Africa and that the majority of victims will be between 15 and 45 years of age.

DISEASE AND DISABILITY IN THE OVER 60S IN INDIA
• Cardiovascular disease commonest cause of death in old age
• 11 million elderly blind people—80% due to cataract
• 60% have hearing impairment
• 9 million have hypertension
• 5 million have diabetes
• 0.35 million have cancer
• 4 million have mental health problems

Table 1.4 WHO report *Ageing in India*, 1999.

Social aspects of ageing

Old age is unfortunately often a time of loss. The potential losses are very varied but are often interrelated, and those that accompany old age are of:

- Health due to increasing pathology.
- Wealth due to termination of employment.
- Companionship following bereavement.
- Independence due to acquired disabilities.
- Homoeostasis due to impairments to autonomic nervous system and renal function.
- Status following retirement and loss of independence.

The above changes and losses may expose the elderly person to the following consequences:

- Unhappiness, grief, depression, suicide (see Chapters 4 and 16).
- Increased incidence of illness.
- Increased risk of accident.
- Poverty.
- Dependence and abuse.
- Malnutrition and subnutrition.
- Hypothermia (see Chapter 12).

Loss of wealth

Income falls on giving up paid employment. Pensions are not normally equivalent to wages and the average pension is approximately 50% of the average working wage for a couple. Disabilities themselves may result in additional costs, e.g. for help, aids and adaptations.

The elderly spend a much higher percentage of their total expenditure on essentials, e.g. heating, food and housing, and there is little opportunity to economize. In the UK, the safety net provided by the social security system is complex and difficult and this alone acts as a deterrent to taking up available benefits. Occupational pensions and investment income are increasing in importance, but in the UK 50% of pensioners receive 75% of their income from the state pension.

Retirement

Retirement is a mixed blessing: 20% of workers fear retirement but 50% look forward to it. Retirement is a potential period of loss — of income, status, companionship and self-confidence.

To counteract the disadvantages, there are the following positive aspects of retirement:

- It may occupy one-third of life.
- Many remain fit and healthy for most of this time.
- It is an opportunity to redesign lifestyle and to promote good health.
- Time is available for new or renewed interests, activities and relationships.

But retirement may bring social problems of its own and it is a time when some difficult decisions will have to be made. Dilemmas encountered may include the following:

- Becoming a carer, e.g. of parents or grandchildren early in retirement or spouse or siblings later on.
- Where to live — it is probably best to stay put where comfortable and well known. If a move is contemplated, earlier is better than later, as the retiree is likely to be fitter and one of a pair.
- What sort of accommodation? Somewhere where independence is possible, even in spite of acquired disabilities.
- Driving — may need to be given up at some stage, so beware of geographical isolation (see Chapters 5 and 16).
- Sex — it is 'allowed' even in very old age so long as it gives pleasure to both partners (see Chapter 13).
- Boredom affects 10% of the retired — another 20% (although not bored) would prefer still to be working. The poor, the disabled, the poorly educated and the isolated are most likely to be dissatisfied with retirement.
- The economic consequences of an expanding population of retired persons dependent on pensions is causing considerable worldwide concern within the developed world. As a consequence, the retirement age may well be gradually increased to 70+ years. In addition, there will also be a need to review the nature of paid employment in later years with consideration of plans to make partial or gradual retirement easier without loss of status, pay or pension rights. Preparation for retirement is vital.

• The increasing frailty and unpredictability of the global financial markets also pose threats to pension provision. The pension aspirations of many current workers may not be met and may be considered a potential threat to world finance.

Recommended physical activity in retirement

• Regular moderate intensity activity for 30 min on most days.
• Short bursts of exertion may have a cumulative effect.
• Start slow and gradually build up intensity and duration.
• If an activity is not provoking symptoms, it is unlikely to be doing harm.
• Generally benefits of activity outweigh risks.
• When activity requires special equipment or clothing, make sure it is appropriate and in good condition.

Some myths of ageing

• *It is a new problem.* No—there have always been elderly people, there are now just more of them. In the past, most people were denied the opportunity of old age by dying young. Now, most babies born in the developed countries can expect to survive into their 80s.
• *All elderly people are decrepit and senile.* No—most live independent lives and mainly in their own homes (96% in the UK).
• *The chronic conditions of old age are untreatable.* No—medical treatment for all ages concerns itself primarily with the management of chronic conditions. The courses of disease can be slowed or modified—e.g. Parkinson's disease or senile dementia of the Alzheimer type—and symptoms can be alleviated—e.g. pain, breathlessness and in deficiency diseases (pernicious anaemia, osteomalacia and myxoedema) normal function can be restored.

• *Natural decline cannot be prevented.* No—regular physical activity in old age can rejuvenate and physical capacity can be improved by 10–15 years. Also, the adoption of a 'healthy lifestyle' in middle age (no smoking, avoidance of obesity and taking regular exercise) can delay the onset and decrease the eventual severity and duration of disability towards the end of life.
• *Treating elderly patients is a waste of money.* No—not to treat is not only inhumane (see Human Rights Act 1998) but often expensive and neglected problems may lead to longer term, higher expenditure (i.e. 'care' can be more expensive than 'cure').
• *Care of the elderly is bankrupting the NHS.* No—it is true that elderly people account for more costs within the NHS than the young (except for the management of children). However, most people make few demands on the NHS until the 15 years prior to their death. Costs for this terminal period are similar if death occurs at any age, i.e. 40 years, 50 years, 60 years, etc. In fact, death in very old age may be gentle and not incur the high cost of unrealistic heroics.
• *All elderly people are depressed and lonely, and are better off dead.* No—the majority of elderly people are not depressed. In fact, well being and contentment may feature in later life more than during the ambitious and frustrated productive years. Although the general population thinks that 90% of elderly people are lonely, only 10% of the elderly consider themselves to be so.
• *The elderly are of no use.* No—they are a valuable resource with experience and, sometimes, wisdom. The majority of carers are elderly and these include grandparents assisting in the rearing of their grandchildren because of absent or working parents. The old are the backbone of the voluntary services.
• *Old patients have a limited future and poor prognosis.* No—life expectancy at 65 years is in excess of 15 years. Survival for 5 years after many surgical and oncological treatments is recorded as a success.

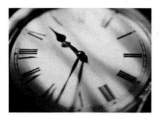

Health and Social Services Care for Elderly People in the UK

Where do elderly people (aged over 65 years) live in the UK?

• In the 'community' — 96%.
• In institutions — 4%; rises to 12% aged over 75 years and 25% over 85 years.

Housing (Table 2.1)

• In the UK the largest housing category is owner-occupiers and accounts for about 60%.
• A high percentage of elderly people (compared with the young) are in rented accommodation — about one-third in council property and half as many in the private sector.
• Elderly people have a higher share of poor housing; the old tend to live in the oldest housing; almost half of the unfit housing in the UK (e.g. lacking one basic amenity, such as inside WC, bath, shower, hot-water supply) is occupied by persons over the age of 65 years.
• Twelve per cent of the elderly population (over 55 years) in the UK live in special accommodation, i.e. purpose-built with warden support (sheltered housing).

Sheltered accommodation

• Originally provided by voluntary organizations and local authority.
• Increasingly now provided by the private sector.
• Consists of purpose-built accommodation for one or two people with built-in aids and adaptations for disabled living and supervised by a warden (who may be on or off site).
• Warden provides support (amount varies from supervision of medication and personal help to just acting as a caller of assistance).
• It is generally too late to move to this type of accommodation once physical and especially mental deterioration has started.
• Development of body-worn alarms means that any housing can be 'sheltered', i.e. help summoned quickly in an emergency.

Community care in the UK

Community care is currently fashionable for the elderly, the mentally ill and the mentally and physically handicapped of all ages. Most elderly people wish to continue to live in their own home but the cost-effectiveness of this is dubious when considerable health or social services support is required. There is also a high social cost to informal carers.

Forty-five per cent of elderly women and 17% of elderly men live alone — the percentage rises for both sexes with increasing age (Table 2.2). In

HOUSING	
Category	%
Owner-occupier	60
Rented from council	24
Sheltered—private	6
Sheltered—council	6
Other	4

Table 2.1 Housing categories of retired people in the UK over 55 years of age. (Source: British Gas Survey, 1990, London.)

ELDERLY PEOPLE LIVING ALONE						
	Men			Women		
Age	1971	1981	1991	1971	1981	1991
65–69	9.07	11.9	14.7	28.4	30.0	29.4
70–74	12.8	16.3	16.9	35.7	39.8	39.7
75–79	16.8	19.2	21.8	40.6	49.5	51.7
80–84	18.8	26.8	28.7	39.1	50.8	55.2
85+	20.3	28.8	32.1	30.0	41.9	48.8

Table 2.2 Per cent of elderly people living alone. (Source: OPCS.)

all, one-third of pensioners live alone; half of them live with their spouses and only one-fifth live with children or siblings or friends. The multiple generation (extended family) is rare in the UK and probably has always been so.

The local authority is the agency responsible for assessing and purchasing community care for residents in their locality. Good community care is essential for the general well-being of most elderly people. Ninety-six per cent of the elderly population live independently, but about 10% of these will require formal community services in order to maintain their independence within their own homes. In the UK, community care continues to be hindered by the split responsibility between the NHS and the local authority for the provision of services to elderly people. The necessary services are multiple and complex (see Table 2.3).

The Community Care Act 1990 attempted to correct the worst deficiencies of the system. The aim of the Act was to maintain elderly people in their own homes for as long as possible and to remove any perverse incentives to admission to institutional care. There has been a reduction in admissions to care homes, but the

targeting of the available domiciliary care to those in greatest need has demoralized many with lesser needs and denied them early and modest interventions which might preserve independence for longer. The later admission of residents to care homes has increased the dependency of care home clients and further stressed the over-stretched staff, who generally remain under-trained and poorly paid.

The setting up of the National Care Standards Commission from April 2002 will hope to improve the situation in care homes and begin to regulate private and voluntary domiciliary care agencies. The regulation of services will no longer be the responsibility of the local authority (previously for residential care homes) or the NHS (previously for nursing homes). The new arrangements will cover wider responsibilities and larger geographical areas (UK regions) and will attempt to introduce national standards throughout the country. The regulatory teams will incorporate staff and members with wider and more expert knowledge than has previously been the case.

The funding of community care remains a serious problem. The local authority remains the

LONG-TERM CARE SERVICES

Domiciliary care		No. of recipients
Home care		610 000
Community nursing		530 000
Day care		260 000
Private help		670 000
Meals		240 000
Institutional care		
Residential care	Publicly financed	205 000
	Privately financed	83 750
	Total	**288 750**
Nursing home care	Publicly financed	115 000
	Privately financed	42 500
	Total	**157 500**
Hospital		**34 000**
All institutional residents		**482 250**

Table 2.3 Number of people in the UK receiving long-term care services by type of service and funding. (Source: PSSRU estimates. *With Respect to Old Age* (1999) p. 9.)

lead agency and has always had the power to charge for its services. Charging policies vary between local authorities, but generally costs are being pushed onto the users (the disabled elderly people). The National Care Standards Commission will also attempt to standardize charging policies. These charging policies cause variable distress and hardship, particularly in regard to high-cost activities, such as care in a residential or nursing home. Means testing is becoming more established and, currently, residents in care homes with capital in excess of £18 500 will get no financial help from the state in meeting their care home fees. About one-third of residents are self-funding and many find it necessary to sell their former home to finance their care. The resulting sale of about 40 000 houses annually within the UK for this purpose caused public disquiet. This was one of the prime reasons for the setting up of the Royal Commission on Long Term Care (see box below). The Commission completed its work quickly and on time, but the government delayed releasing the report and refused to follow all its recommendations. The most significant deviations from the recommendations concern the financing of per-

sonal care. The Royal Commission recommended that this, like nursing care, should be free at the time of use. The government has refused this for England, but the devolved assembly of Scotland has not.

Report by the Royal Commission on Long Term Care—March 1999 (with respect to old age)

Main recommendations
- The cost of care for those individuals who need it should be split between living costs, housing costs and personal care. Personal care should be available after an assessment according to need and paid for from general taxation; the rest should be subject to a co-payment according to means.
- The government should establish a National Care Commission which would monitor longitudinal trends including demography and spending, ensure transparency and accountability in the system, represent the interest of consumers, encourage innovation, keep under review the market for residential care, nursing care and national benchmarks now and in the future.

National Service Framework for Older People

This was published in March 2001. It is one of a series of 'frameworks' and was prepared by a multi-disciplinary committee set up by the government to improve standards within the statutory services. It provides recommendations provided by both the NHS and local authority social services departments. It concerns standards of care for elderly people, both in hospital and in their own homes and pays particular attention to conditions such as stroke and falls, which particularly affect the older members of our population.

Recommendations of the National Service Framework for Older People

• *Standard 1 — routing out age discrimination.* NHS services will be provided regardless of age on the basis of clinical need alone. Social care services will not use age in their eligibility criteria or policies to restrict access to available services. Ageism is, however, often covert rather than explicit.

• *Standard 2 — person centred care.* NHS and social care services will treat older people as individuals and enable them to make choices about their own care. This is achieved through the single assessment process, integrated commissioning arrangement, and integrated provision of services including community equipment and continence services.

• *Standard 3 — intermediate care.* Older people will have access to a new range of intermediate care services at home or in designated care settings to promote their independence by providing enhanced services from the NHS and local councils to prevent unnecessary hospital admission, effective rehabilitation services to enable early discharge from hospital, and to prevent premature or unnecessary admission to long-term residential care.

• *Standard 4 — general hospital care.* Older people's care in hospital is delivered through appropriate specialist care and by hospital staff who have the right set of skills to meet their needs.

• *Standard 5 — stroke.* The NHS will take action to prevent stroke, working in partnership with other agencies where appropriate.

• *Standard 6 — falls.* The NHS, working in partnership with councils, will take action to prevent falls and reduce resultant fractures or other injuries in their populations of older people.

• *Standard 7 — mental health in older people.* Older people who have mental health problems will have access to integrated mental health services provided by the NHS and councils to ensure effective diagnosis, treatment and support for them and their carers.

• *Standard 8 — the promotion of health and active life in older age.* The health and well-being of older people is promoted through a co-ordinated programme of action led by the NHS with support from councils.

Who cares?

Informal carers

These are the most important members of the caring workforce. They are unpaid, untrained, but devoted and effective. Although the generations tend to live apart, there continues to be frequent contact within a family and almost 50% of elderly people living alone have regular daily contact with a family member. The bulk of community support is provided by family and friends ('informal carers') — the following points are relevant to the situation within the UK.

• The proportion of dependants, i.e. children under 16 years, men over 65 years and women over 60 years of age in the community, has not increased during this century (Table 2.4).

• There are now more dependent elderly people in the community than dependent children.

• It is calculated that in the UK there are 6 million informal carers.

• Most carers are women (60%) and over half of 'housewives' can expect to be called upon at some time to help an elderly and infirm person.

• Many carers are themselves pensioners. The mean age of carers of confused elderly people is 61 years.

DEPENDANTS

Year	%
1901	41
1951	37
1981	40
1991	39
2001	40

Table 2.4 Percentage of dependants in the community, i.e. pensioners and children.

Needs of carers

Recognition
• By family and friends
• By professionals
• By the state
Support
• Financial
• Social
• Psychological
• Professional
• Self-help groups
Respite
• Short periods (e.g. day care)
• Long periods — intermittent admission to care
• Sitting services
• Immediate in emergencies
Information
• About the patient's illness
• About available services

Statutory services

The so-called statutory services are provided in combination by the local authority, which is financed through the Council Tax, and by the NHS staff, who are funded by central government. Increasingly the local authority services are delegated to private and voluntary organizations, who act as agents. Services may be obtained by application to the departments of social services or through the primary health-care team. They may be free or a charge may be made. Most NHS services are provided free of charge and are arranged through the patient's registered GP. Where NHS charges do exist, there is usually exemption for people of pensionable age or financial assistance can be obtained. The National Standards Care Commission (see above) will attempt to unify charges and standards.

Local authority services

Home-care services — local authority and independent sector
Domiciliary care services
These are the linchpin of organized community support. They initially started as a domestic service with the provision of help with cleaning but gradually expanded to cover cooking, shopping and, increasingly, personal care. Visits by the home-care assistant may range from a few hours per week up to three or more visits a day, depending on needs and availability. The number of staff has not kept up with demographic trends. Private schemes are now developing in the UK but provision is patchy and regulation variable. As the service now concentrates on personal care, the domestic cleaning services are increasingly being taken over by voluntary organizations and the private sector.

Meals-on-wheels service
This provides clients with hot meals in their own home.
• Meals are provided at mid-day, usually just two or three times per week.
• There are great practical problems in providing meals which remain appetizing and nutritious after delays caused by preparation, storage and delivery.

• Alternative methods of providing a regular meal service have been tried, e.g. frozen meals, which require reheating, and boil-in-the-bag prepared meals. Many in need are too disabled to cope with such systems.

• If mainly dependent on meals on wheels for nutrition, more than four meals per week are required to fulfil the recommended minimal dietary requirements.

• Currently in the UK more than 26 million meals are provided by this service each year and about 3% of elderly people benefit, rising to 12% in the over-85s.

Luncheon clubs

These are centres where meals are provided, usually at subsidized prices, run by either the local authority or voluntary organizations. They provide meals to 3% of the elderly population, i.e. similar provision to meals-on-wheels service. Frequency of meal provision from luncheon clubs is less than that provided by the meals-on-wheels service — usually just once or twice weekly — but companionship is offered in addition to food. Transport is often a limiting factor.

Day centres

These are very varied and may be run by the local authority or voluntary groups and must not be confused with day hospitals. Staff may be trained (social workers, therapists) or untrained or a combination of both. A charge for attendance is usually made and transport may be provided. About 5% of elderly people attend day centres.

The aims of day centres

• To combat loneliness
• To provide diversional activity and recreation
• To provide a meal and other comforts
• To relieve other supporters
• To introduce clients to other forms of care
• To disseminate health education, etc.

NHS community services

Primary health care in the future in the UK will be provided through Primary Care Trusts. These will serve populations up to one-third of a million people. They will employ all medical, nursing and allied professions (but not social service employees) who work in the community. They will be expected to work in conjunction with the local authority social services departments. They will also be responsible for commissioning the services provided by their local hospitals and play an important part in planning local health services through Health Improvement Plans (HImPs) and joint planning with the local authority and hospital services.

General practitioners

In the UK every person is registered with a GP, who acts as the first point of contact for all NHS services. If multidisciplinary care is to succeed in the community setting, it is essential that the GP becomes the effective leader of the team. The good GP needs:

• A wide knowledge of both medicine and the scope of the skills of the other team members.
• Comprehensive records detailing the patient's past medical history.
• Up-to-date information about the patient's current problems and treatment.
• A friendly and approachable manner so that neither elderly patients nor their carers (formal or informal) are deterred from seeking help.
• Ready access to hospital-based specialists' help and advice.

General practitioners who wish to demonstrate their special interest and skills in managing the health problems of elderly people can do so by passing the Diploma of Geriatric Medicine examination of the Royal College of Physicians.

Anticipatory care in the community

In general practice in the UK there are many potential opportunities for doctors to prevent illness and promote improved health in elderly people. An age/gender register is essential for such activities.

Potentially preventable diseases in old age

- Multi-infarct dementia and stroke by treatment of BP and anticoagulation for atrial fibrillation
- Osteoporosis by hormone-replacement therapy in post-menopausal women and by exercise
- Ischaemic heart disease by avoidance of tobacco and dietary change
- Alcoholic dementia, heart failure, pancreatitis and cirrhosis
- Obesity and its effect on osteoarthritis and carbohydrate metabolism
- Diverticular disease and gall-bladder disease by increasing dietary fibre
- Chronic obstructive airways disease and bronchogenic carcinoma, risks reduced by tobacco abstinence
- Dietary deficiency states
- Iatrogenic disease

Opportunistic case finding

During any consultation the opportunity should be taken to pick up on other health or social problems.

Community nursing staff

Community nurses

Eighty per cent of the total time of these nurses is devoted to the care of elderly people. They provide:

- Hands-on nursing.
- Treatment, e.g. injections, enemas and dressings.
- Specialist care, e.g. stoma management and continence advice.
- Liaison with other services.

Health visitors

Only 15% of their time is devoted to the care of the elderly and, at present, their involvement with this age-group appears to be declining. However, they play a valuable role in that they:

- Advise, counsel and educate.
- Identify needs.

- Practise prevention.
- Liaise with other services.

Community psychiatric nurses

This is a small but expanding group of community workers and their main tasks are:

- To support the patients and carers.
- To monitor progress or deterioration.
- To liaise with other services.

NB: All community nurses require specialist training in community needs and techniques. The nursing staff may be augmented by less specialized aides and informal carers.

Institutional care

This is available and necessary for only a minority of elderly people (4% in the UK). The number of local authority homes has decreased over recent years, while the independent sector (mainly private) has expanded, encouraged by the availability of state benefits and lack of control over entry requirements (Table 2.5). It may now be contracting again as local authorities are unable to provide realistic funding. The proportion of elderly people in care is much higher in other Western countries than in the UK (Table 2.6).

Reasons for institutionalization

- Severe physical disabilities.
- Immobile without help.
- Severe mental disabilities, constant supervision needed.
- Passive/dependent personality.
- Hostile community or non-existent community support.
- Unpredictable and frequent care needs.
- Wealth makes choice possible between community and institutional care.

NB: Usually at least two criteria are required in the UK to qualify for care in the public sector.

Complications of institutionalization

- Depersonalization.
- Marked restriction of choices.
- Accelerated dependence.

NB: All of these can be minimized by persistent effort by residents and staff.

LONG-TERM CARE PROVISION

	1983	1994
Total no. long-term care places	280 000	465 000
NHS places	55 600 (20)	37 500 (8)
Private/voluntary nursing homes	18 200 (6.5)	148 500 (32)
Local authority residential homes	115 900 (41.5)	68 900 (15)
Voluntary residential homes	37 600 (13)	45 500 (10)
Private residential homes	51 800 (19)	164 200 (35)

Percentage of total in parentheses.

Table 2.5 Changes in long-term care provision in the UK.

NURSING HOME USAGE

	Example
Low 4% or less	UK (4%)
Medium 5–6%	USA (5.7%)
High >7%	The Netherlands (10.9%)

Table 2.6 Nursing home usage by people over the age of 65 years.

Residential care

In the UK this is provided by both the local authority and the private sector — but there is no uniformity of geographical availability.

Most residents on entry are now over 80 years of age and suffer from multiple disabilities (both physical and mental (Table 2.7)) and need both 'hotel services' and help with personal hygiene.

Medical cover is provided by the resident's own GP and, if nursing help is required for specific tasks, this is provided by the community nursing staff as if the patient were still living in his or her own home. The permanent staff of the home will be either residential social workers or care assistants — other specialist help may be available on demand from the usual domiciliary services. If disabilities become more severe, a move to a nursing home may be needed.

Long-term care

Responsibility has now been switched in the UK to the local authority. Charges are made (means

tested) for most services — especially nursing and residential care homes. There is much anxiety about future provision and costs, the individual being responsible for board and lodging and, in England, 'personal' care but not nursing is subject to means-testing. Owner-occupiers often therefore have to sell to finance care unless a dependent relative continues to live in the house or insurance arrangements have been made.

A small number of free NHS continuing-care beds remain available, but with very strict entry criteria (eligibility criteria), which are fixed locally and show considerable variability. Only the most severely disabled are eligible and those with an anticipated short prognosis.

Respite care (for relief of informal carers) is also now mainly the responsibility of the local authority social services department.

Care home care

The UK care home sector is faced with the following problems:

DISABILITY IN CARE

	Local authority residential home	Private residential home	Voluntary residential home	Private nursing home	NHS geriatric beds	NHS psychogeriatric bed
Unable to walk alone	9%	17%		50%	86%	31%
Mentally impaired	52%		50%	66%	80%	91%
Incontinent urine	17%	18%		35%	71%	57%
Incontinent faeces	16%	15%	28%	55%	63%	

Table 2.7 Disability in care (west Glasgow). (*Source:* D.J. Stott *et al.* (1990) Functional capacity and mental status of elderly people in long-term care in west Glasgow. *Health Bulletin* 48, 17–24.)

1 Increasing numbers of old old (i.e. those over 85 years of age).
2 Increasing frailty of residents — especially dementia with behavioural problems.
3 Inadequate budgets.
4 Staff recruitment and retention problems.
5 Financial consequences of increasing staff numbers and improving staff training and pay.
6 Rising public aspirations and expectations.
7 Falling numbers of available beds.
8 The demands of recent legislation regarding space.

Respite care

This is the temporary provision of a bed in a care home or hospital for frail patients with chronic degenerative diseases, where all hope of achieving improvement or reversal of changes have been abandoned, in order to allow the informal carers to enjoy a well-earned break.

Periods of respite care often have an adverse effect on the recipient — especially if they are unable to comprehend the reasons and needs for such respite care.

Respite care should not be confused with crisis intervention, i.e. when a supporting system suddenly collapses, nor should it be considered as top-up rehabilitation. The latter is a separate function and should be provided in a rehabilitation setting and on a planned and regular basis.

Rehabilitation and intermediate care

Principles of rehabilitation

1 Rehabilitation is needed after all illnesses not just after stroke or fracture, etc.
2 It is a multi-disciplinary activity including the patient and the patient's informal carers.
3 A full assessment of the patient's problems are required before the process starts.
4 Goals must be realistic with defined end-points.
5 There must be a logical step-by-step approach to achieve the set goals.
6 It is a continuous process — 'every activity is a therapeutic opportunity', i.e. rehabilitation does not just occur when face to face with a therapist.
7 Rehabilitation should never really end as maintenance is required if the achieved improvements are to be retained.
8 Rehabilitation can take place in a variety of settings depending on circumstances.

THE REHABILITATION TEAM

Patient
Family
Voluntary workers
Clinical psychologist
Chiropodist
Nurses and health visitors
Rehabilitation professions (physiotherapists, occupational
    therapists, speech therapists)
Appliance officer
Social worker
Doctor

Table 2.8

9 Rehabilitation is not always the most appropriate way to manage severe disability. A palliative approach is sometimes the best and kindest option.

Barriers to successful rehabilitation
- Global impairment of higher cerebral function.
- Poor motivation (patient or carers).
- Depression.
- Communication difficulties.
- Sensory deprivation.
- Associated pathology (arthritis, heart failure).
- Pressure sores, contractures.
- Loss of body image, sensory ataxia, disordered visuospatial perception.
- Swallowing difficulty.
- Unrealistic expectations.
- Effects of disease, injury, etc.

Rehabilitation
Rehabilitation is defined as the restoration of the individual to his or her fullest physical, mental and social capability. It takes several forms:

1 Restoration to full activity after a severe illness (e.g. abdominal surgery, myocardial infarction).

2 Restoration of maximum achievable function following a specific impairment (e.g. stroke, fractured femoral neck).

3 Facilitating the achievement of as much independence as possible despite continuing impairment (e.g. Parkinson's disease, amputation, partially recovered stroke, hip disease).

Rehabilitation is carried out by members of the rehabilitation team (Table 2.8) in a variety of settings (Table 2.9).

- Impairment—loss or abnormality of structure or function, e.g. weak leg and arm following stroke.
- Disability—the resulting loss of ability to perform an activity in the normal manner, e.g. a diminished ability to walk.
- Handicap—the ensuing disadvantage in terms of fulfilment of the individual's role, e.g. unable to cook and do the housework, participate in leisure activities, etc.

Rehabilitation from acute illness
Hospital admission is often required, not for specific investigations or medication that cannot be administered at home, but because the weakness associated with a chest infection or heart disease renders patients unable to attend to their bodily needs (nutrition, fluid intake, bowel, bladder, hygiene, etc.) unassisted. He or she may feel too unwell to get out of bed for a day or two. Unless there is adequate support at home, admission needs to be arranged without delay, otherwise pressure sores, contractures, constipation, incontinence and loss of confidence are inevitable and will necessitate protracted rehabilitation. Remobilization is achieved by suitable exercises (passive, assisted, resisted), combined with functional exercise,

REHABILITATION SITES

Acute hospital ward (includes orthopaedic wards)
Rehabilitation ward in acute hospital
Rehabilitation ward in community hospital
Stroke units, wherever situated
Outpatient therapy departments
Geriatric day hospital
Psychiatric counterparts of the above
Primary-care premises
Residential/nursing homes
Keep-fit classes, stroke clubs, etc.
Patients' own homes (e.g. domiciliary therapy, patients' and
    carers' own efforts)

Table 2.9 Where does rehabilitation take place?

such as transfers, sitting to standing, and walking. Activities of daily living (ADL) abilities are assessed and various items of equipment may be deployed to facilitate independence. An attempt at quantitative measurement of function is provided by the Barthel scale (see Appendix 2). Following discharge, the able-bodied may consider positive measures to promote physical fitness.

Intermediate care

This is described in Standard 3 of the National Service Framework (see above). It covers many aspects of the management of frail elderly patients. It is expected to help maintain elderly people in the community and to avoid hospital admission by intensifying care provision at times of need (e.g. an acute minor illness), to aid recovery by the provision by rehabilitation services, to assist the discharge of elderly patients from hospital through active rehabilitation programmes and to enhance the domiciliary support at the time of discharge (and is in danger of being all things to all men).

Intermediate care therefore has a role in community care, i.e. enhanced provision, and also in hospital care in the form of rehabilitation and step-down care. This latter is envisaged as a less intense, more user friendly, less clinical, more domestic provision of inpatient services. In many ways, it plans to replace what was previously described as slow-stream hospital rehabilitation. Some of the provision may be nurse-led, moving away from the more doctor-led medical model. However, those receiving intermediate care are likely to be very frail and vulnerable to repeated episodes of deterioration in their health, and the input of geriatricians is essential. The current NHS modernization plan proposes the provision of an additional 7000 intermediate care beds within the next few years.

Day hospitals

These are units that provide day treatment to patients living in their own homes. Both psychogeriatric and geriatric patients are catered for, but usually separately. Transport has always been problematic. Day hospitals are capable of providing all the services available to inpatients, i.e. respite, rehabilitation, diagnosis, investigation, monitoring of medication and even continuing care. Unfortunately, the latter activity has gained many day hospitals a reputation for becoming stagnant and undynamic units and has played a role in the demise of day hospitals. Hopefully lessons have been learnt and with the reprovision of finances for intermediate care, the day hospital may be due for a renaissance as it was a successful method of avoiding admission, shortening inpatient stays and providing extra post-discharge support after inpatient care.

Scale of disability in old age

- 11% of elderly men over 65 years are disabled
- 90% of elderly women over 65 years are disabled
- 1.3 million elderly individuals are disabled
- 38% of disabled elderly people are over the age of 85 years
- 80% of elderly disabled people need help at least once a day
- 63% of disabled elderly people use acute hospitals within a 2-year period (43% as inpatients)
- 38% of disabled elderly people have cognitive impairment
- 29% of physically disabled elderly people use formal community services

Provision of aids and adaptations

This activity is mainly the responsibility of the local authority, except for the provision of prostheses such as hearing aids, artificial limbs etc. which are provided by the National Health Service. Delays in assessment and provision are frequent and many of the items and services provided are not always appropriate to the patient's needs.

UK hospital care of elderly patients

This takes the following forms:

1 Outpatient care, i.e. accident and emergency attendance and outpatient clinics.
2 Acute inpatient care.
3 Intermediate care/rehabilitation care.
4 Long-term care.

Outpatient care

Accident and emergency departments

Because of their liability to accidents, and the sudden and unexpected onset of illness, the elderly are great users of the accident and emergency (A & E) department. Unfortunately, their management in such departments is difficult and the outcome sub-optimal. The follow-

ing points are some of the reasons for these difficulties.

1 Elderly patients are often unable to give an account of themselves due to changing level of consciousness, confusion or dementia, communication difficulties (speech, hearing impairment), anxiety or fear.
2 Their problems are frequently multiple and complex.
3 They are often unaccompanied.
4 Their accident or incident is often a consequence of long-term neglect or lack of support.
5 They wait longer to be seen, take longer to be admitted and longer to be discharged than younger patients.
6 They are more likely than most patients to require transport back home.

An overnight ward as part of the A & E department may allow sufficient time for the elderly to regain their equilibrium and for intermediate care in the community to be organized and thereby facilitate discharge and enhance their post-discharge support.

The department of geriatric medicine should have sufficient experienced staff to provide an immediate 24 h per day expert advisory service to their local A & E department.

Outpatient department

- Irrespective of age, all appropriate patients have a right to be referred to any specialist clinic.
- Frail elderly patients are more likely to require assistance with transport to the hospital and within the hospital.
- All clinics should be user-friendly for elderly patients; e.g. variable height couches, effective arrangements for deaf or partially sighted patients in the waiting area and arrangements to communicate with deaf patients (e.g. an available and working communicator). Help with dressing and undressing is also likely to be needed.
- Complex patients with multiple pathology are best co-ordinated by specialist geriatric clinics, supported where necessary by organ-specific specialists.
- Follow-up clinics where necessary should be

held near to the patient's home, e.g. GP surgery or community hospital and not necessarily at the district general hospital.

Acute inpatient care

During the last 20 years, the acute bed numbers in British hospitals have been reduced by 2% annually, although this process may now be reversed. At the same time, admissions have risen by 3.5–5%. The elderly are the greatest users of hospital beds (65% of inpatients are over 65 years of age). Occupancy rates have always been high and often reach 97%. The system has only continued to function by the steady reduction in the length of stay for each patient including the elderly.

Most admissions are considered appropriate with between 1% and 6% being deemed not so. Inappropriate admission may be higher amongst older patients, perhaps up to 20%, especially in the very old. However, the rates of inappropriate admissions are very variable and depend on the quality of local general practices and the availability of alternative forms of care.

Reasons which expose elderly people to higher hospital admission rates are:
1 Pathology, both acute and chronic.
2 Living alone and social disadvantage.
3 Polypharmacy.
4 High accident/fall rate.
5 Repeated admissions (the 'revolving door').
The last should not automatically be considered as a failure. Recurrent short admission of exacerbations or deterioration in long-term illnesses may be the most appropriate way of coping with chronic conditions. This ensures that the patient spends as many days as possible in his or her own home if that is his or her wish.

If the new concept of intermediate care is successful, it may make some admissions unnecessary and shorten those that are—we watch with interest.

Hospital hazards

The acute hospital is a particularly dangerous place for frail elderly people. This is not a reason for depriving them of access, but should act as a stimulus to improving the safety of patients through better hospital design, improved staffing levels and mix and improving standards of cleanliness and catering.

• Up to 50% of deaths of elderly patients in hospital are said to be precipitated by poor prescribing.

• Ten per cent of all hospital inpatients suffer from cross-infections, especially with MRSA. This rate is highest and most dangerous in frail elderly people.

• Broad-spectrum antibiotics may precipitate bowel overgrowth by *Clostridium difficile* and the resulting diarrhoea that may have fatal consequences.

• Falls are common because of impaired function in the patient or hospital design and inadequate staff supervision. The situation is often made worse by the inappropriate use of various forms of restraint (both physical and pharmacological).

• Patients who are malnourished on admission may deteriorate further in their nutritional status during their hospital stay due to inappropriate catering and feeding arrangements.

• Dependency may be encouraged by poor staff attitudes and practices.

• Elderly patients are not always given appropriate priority when investigations are needed. Subsequent delays can be very detrimental. Sophisticated techniques may be more appropriate because of the elderly patient's inability to cope with demanding and invasive techniques as well as their fitter and younger counterparts.

• Surgery is more dangerous, especially if delegated to junior surgeons and anaesthetists.

• Malnutrition hampers surgical recovery.

• Ignoring pre- and post-operative medical conditions compromises the success of essential surgery.

• Post-operative complications are more common and more serious.

• Lack of appropriate community services and/or accommodation may delay discharge. Up to 70 000 patients are trapped in this way in UK hospitals at any one time. These inappropriately labelled bed-blockers or delayed discharges continue to be exposed to all of the above dangers and occupy about 6% of acute hospital beds.

The department of geriatric medicine

This should provide the ideal setting for the medical and nursing management of frail elderly patients with multiple and complex problems. It should be based within the district general hospital, but with out-reach facilities in more peripheral (?community) hospitals, the community itself and care homes. In addition, it should provide advice and support for other hospital departments caring for elderly patients, especially orthopaedic surgery and psychiatry.

Admission to a department of geriatric medicine should not deprive but hasten access to other specialist opinions, such as cardiology, neurology, etc.

NHS continuing care

This service no longer exists in all health districts as some have contracted out all such activity to local nursing homes.

Where NHS continuing care beds still function, they are usually few in number and only accessed through strict eligibility criteria such as:
• Very heavy dependency levels needing frequent specialist nursing and medical supervision.
• Where expensive equipment is required that is not usually available within a nursing home.
• Where the patient's prognosis is likely to be shorter than the time needed to arrange a transfer to accommodation in the independent sector.
• Where the independent sector refuses to accept responsibility for a patient's care on the basis of complexity, lack of specialist staffing and facilities or where anticipated costs are not going to be covered by the standard funding made available through the statutory authorities.

Financial allowances which can be claimed by some UK pensioners

1 Basic state pension plus Christmas bonus plus winter fuel payments. The basic state pension is provided when the necessary fulfilment of national insurance contributions has been made during working life. A single person's pension in 2001/02 was £72.50. A married couple during the same year could receive between £115.90–£145.00 depending on national insurance contributions previously made. Graduated or additional contributions may be made towards the pension if appropriate contributions had been made in earlier years. Pensions are not reduced if the person continues to work beyond 65 years for men and 60 years for women.
2 Income support—savings must be minimal. Value of home not included, but any other properties must be taken into account.

Grounds for possible extra money—usually for people receiving income support

• Age over 80
• Blindness
• Mortgage interest
• Water rates
• Ground rent and service charges
• House insurance and repairs
• Special diet
• Bereavement
• Special laundry, e.g. for incontinence
• Heating, e.g. cold weather payments and help with insulation work
• Hospital fares and other special transport costs
• Board and lodging for residential care and nursing homes
• Council tax

3 Social fund (community care grants). Loans made for replacement of clothing, repairs to home, redecoration, bedding and furniture, etc.
4 Housing benefit from the local authority housing department for rent.

5 Attendance allowance (day or night allowances) routinely only paid for disabilities of greater duration than 6 months, but payment may be accelerated during a terminal illness. Non-means tested and paid to the claimant. Help with bodily functions or high intensity attendance has to be demonstrated.

6 Extra money for carers.

(a) Invalid care allowance for a carer who is a low wage earner and who provides more than 35 h of care per week and is aged under 65 years.

(b) Home responsibility protection to protect pension rights of carers.

7 Death grant to help pay for funerals if extra financial help is required. It must be requested before the funeral is carried out.

8 Concessions are available for all pensioners for bus and rail travel and entry to places of entertainment—but local variations in generosity and age qualifications.

9 All pensioners over the age of 75 are now entitled to a free television licence.

NB: Disabled living allowance including mobility allowance are not available to persons over the age of 65.

Benefits rights services/officers are provided by some local authorities or voluntary organizations, such as the Citizens Advice Bureau, Help the Aged and Age Concern. They provide a free advice service regarding the availability of benefits.

The benefit system is extremely complicated and forever changing. For current details see the Age Concern publication *Your Rights*, which is published annually.

Commission for Health Improvement

The Commission for Health Improvement (CHI), set up by the Department of Health at the end of the 1990s, has the role of monitoring and improving standards in hospital care. This includes elderly patients wherever they are accommodated within a hospital. The plan is for multi-disciplinary teams, which include managers, to regularly review district services and report directly back to the Department of Health. This will assist in the production of league tables, etc. The teams are particularly concerned with matters of hospital governance and audit.

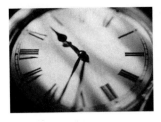

Special Features of Medicine in the Elderly

The ageing of populations

Developed countries experienced a large increase in the proportion of elderly citizens during the 20th century, particularly during its closing decade which saw rising numbers of people in their 80s and 90s. Reasons for this include falling fertility rates and falling death rates at all ages but particularly in infancy and early childhood—due to improved living standards (housing, hygiene, nutrition, heating).

The increasing number of very elderly people in developed countries is, however, partly due to the improvements in curative medicine in adult life. In the UK the 2001 census showed that for the first time, the number of children (age 16 or under) was less than the number of pensioners (women of 60 and over and men of 65 and over).

Many underdeveloped countries are also experiencing a growth in older people, sometimes exaggerated by the loss of the younger generation due to HIV infection.

Blessing or curse?

Increasing longevity sounds like a blessing—but that depends on whether the extra years are years of good health and activity. Does the 'rec-tangularization of the survival curve' lead to a 'compression of morbidity' into the final months of life or to a prolonged period of disability and dependency? One recent estimate gave a 65-year-old man an average of 8 further years of active life followed by 6 years of significant disability, and a woman 10 years and 9 years, respectively. At age 75, these figures were 4 years and 4 years for a man, and 6.5 years and 4.5 years for a woman.

The ageing cell

Some cells (neuronal, renal and myocardial) do not divide and have to last a lifetime, although there is a decline in their numbers. Normal human embryonic fibroblasts have a fixed capacity to divide around 50 times, but those from mature subjects have a reduced capacity for reduplication. This may be due to telomerase inactivation in somatic (unlike germ-line) cells with telomere shortening, telomerase reactivation being a possible explanation for the immortality of malignant cells in culture. Other features of these cells from aged individuals include:
1 Aneuploidy (variable chromosome numbers).
2 Increased numbers of nucleoli.

3 Lipofuscin pigment granules in cytoplasm in neurons, liver, kidney, muscle.
4 Mitochondrial respiratory-chain function (energy release) less efficient in skeletal muscle.
5 Cells are more vulnerable to free-radical damage.

Ageing connective tissue

Stiffness and loss of elasticity occurs due to cross-linkages (e.g. disulphide bonds) forming bridges between adjacent collagen molecules, especially in skin, elastic laminae of blood vessels, tendons and lens of eye.

Immunity and ageing

1 Thymic involution and attenuated T-cell-mediated immunity lead to reactivation of quiescent infections, such as TB and varicella. There seems to be a decline in delayed-type skin-hypersensitivity reactions to injected antigens (anergy) in many frail aged subjects.
2 Certain autoantibodies occur more frequently in old age—e.g. antiphospholipid antibodies, which are associated with vascular disease but their significance in older people is uncertain.
3 Proliferative disorders of the lymphocyte are very common.
4 Malnutrition and diabetes compound these problems.

Declining function

Many physiological parameters decline with age but the magnitude of the decline is hard to estimate. These figures are almost always based on cross-sectional rather than longitudinal studies, which will include individuals within the elderly cohort who have acquired diseases that may affect function—renal function will suffer as a result of hypertension or diabetes, for example—or whose sedentary lifestyle in retirement has caused cardiorespiratory fitness

to decline through disuse. In order to be attributable to ageing *per se*, a phenomenon must be universal, intrinsic and progressive. Watching the London Marathon will reveal many 70- or even 80+-year-olds fitter than most people in their 30s and 40s.

Special features of illness in older patients

Illness in older people is usually a continuum of conditions found in middle age, but the illness occurs in the context of ageing and lack of fitness, and the social situation the person is in (Fig. 3.1).

Background of ageing
Ageing changes are seen in **most organs** (go through the body in your mind), e.g. brain, special senses, peripheral nerves.

Why do ageing changes matter?
• Increased variability between individuals.
• OK at rest, significant when stressed (e.g. fasting glucose minimally higher in elderly, but glucose levels higher after meals).

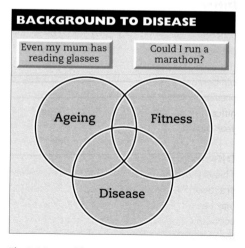

Fig. 3.1 In an older person, the impact of the disease depends on the level of fitness and physiological ageing of the individual.

- Impaired homeostasis results in problems when the environment becomes more challenging. In extreme old age the challenge may be minimal, such as maintaining BP on standing. Some physical signs have different significance, e.g. small pupils, poor upgaze, wasting of small muscles of the hand.

Multiple pathology and aetiology
Why do old people often have several diseases?
The prevalence of many diseases increases with age (e.g. stroke, Parkinson's disease, Alzheimer's disease) so the fact that older people have several diseases may simply reflect this. Some chronic diseases have complications affecting several systems (e.g. diabetes may lead to heart, eye, kidney and nerve problems) or may predispose to other disorders (e.g. infections). Also, a risk factor may predispose to several diseases (e.g. smokers are more likely to have chronic bronchitis, lung cancer, heart disease, strokes, gangrene and osteoporosis). One problem may also have several causes (multiple aetiology); e.g. falls are usually multi-factorial (previous stroke + poor vision + osteoarthritis of the knees, etc).

Different risk factors
It must not be assumed that parameters (e.g. high lipid levels) that constitute a risk factor in the young carry the same risk in the elderly in the absence of positive evidence. An 85-year-old person with a cholesterol level of 8 mmol/L presumably has 'protective' genes and so the significance of this finding is not the same as in a 40-year-old person.

Different susceptibility to disease
This is more of a theoretical possibility than a practical consideration. However, tuberculosis may be commoner (reasons may include socio-economic factors, prior exposure, changes in the immune system, etc).

Different differential diagnosis
Although the range of possible diagnoses may be similar at any age, age is important in deter-mining what is most likely. Consider fits and jaundice: the commonest causes will be different in the neonate, child, young adult and old person.

Altered response to disease
Many older people present in exactly the same way as middle-aged people, e.g. crushing central chest pain in a myocardial infarct. However, this is not always the case and this makes diagnosis in the frail older person a diagnostic challenge. There may be:
- Missing symptoms, e.g. pain, fever, thirst.
- Missing signs, e.g. neck stiffness.
   Finally, non-specific presentation is common. The 'geriatric giants'—the big 'I's—are common features of illness in old age:
- Intellectual failure (acute or chronic confusion).
- Incontinence (if this is new, why?).
- Immobility ('off her feet').
- Instability (falls).
- Iatrogenic disease (see below).
- Inability to look after oneself (functional decline or in an analogy to paediatrics, 'failure to thrive').
All of these vague and dull-sounding clinical pictures, often labelled 'social problem' in the notes, are almost never due to social problems and could be due to a huge range of serious and treatable conditions—if you look—e.g. myocardial infarct, PE, stroke, PD, etc.

Consequences of immobility
These include dehydration, incontinence, pressure sores, deep vein thrombosis, etc. and often complicate the presenting condition.

Low expectations
Why do old people sometimes present so late in their illness?
Older people may have poor expectations of the health care sytem fuelled by friends and family and sometimes, sadly, by previous experience of health care professionals. 'What do you expect at your age?' is a remark familiar to many. The problem may be compounded by lack of medical understanding, so that urinary inconti-

nence and swollen ankles are assumed to be normal.

Social problems

Old age is a time of loss (family, friends, income, housing, mobility, independence and life itself). This is one aspect of medicine for older people that can be sad. There may be practical solutions — how will the problems affect the patient? However, often what are most appreciated are support and a little of your time to hear about how things were.

Advantages and disadvantages of 'labels'

Be circumspect before labelling people. Doctors spend a great deal of time attaching diagnostic labels to people. This is part of the job; the label usually helps the patient to understand what is causing their symptoms and helps the clinicians to manage the condition. However, sometimes labels are unhelpful — a 93-year-old woman with impaired glucose tolerance labelled 'diabetic' may be refused Christmas cake in her residential home. It is very difficult to shake off an incorrect label and so if in doubt remain descriptive, e.g. 'breathless with shadow on CXR', pending further investigation.

The importance of functional assessment and rehabilitation

Expensive and technically successful intervention is of limited value if the patient does not recover the ability to enjoy a worthwhile quality of life — hence the importance and interest of multi-disciplinary team working. Overall assessment should include a comprehensive list of medical problems and their prioritization in terms of threat to quality and quantity of life (an assessment of cognitive function, evaluation of functional abilities, some idea of the social background ('ecological niche') and who is there to do tasks for the patient when he or she is unable to do them for him or herself). The Barthel scale attempts to quantify function (see Appendix 2). It will take an older person longer to recover strength and function after a severe systemic illness — this may be obvious to the reader, but is not always obvious to patient, family and medical attendant. Rehabilitation can take place in a variety of settings. It is an active process and it is important that the patient and often the carer share the same objectives as the multi-disciplinary team. Regular goal setting meetings are useful. If the patient is not progressing as well as anticipated it is important to look for barriers that may be interfering with the process. These include depression, uncontrolled pain and hidden agendas, e.g. 'if I improve I will be a burden to them'.

Ethical problems

The whole area of denial of access to high-class care versus over-aggressive and futile intervention — discriminating ageism versus compassionate ageism — is a major minefield and one of the fascinations of geriatric medicine. See also Chapter 16.

Examination of the aged patient — things to look out for

Gait
- Aided or unaided?
- Foot drop?
- Shuffling or striding? Stable or unstable?
- Difficulty up/down from chair?
- Parkinsonian or multi-infarct?

Face
- Parkinsonian (the 'disconcerting reptilian gaze', immobility, flexed posture).
- Depression.
- Hypothyroidism, anaemia, vitiligo.
- Angular stomatitis (often due to ill-fitting dentures).
- Orofacial dyskinesia.
- Ptosis — symmetrical ('senile') or unilateral (eye surgery or pathological).
- Basal-cell carcinoma.
- Facial palsy.

Joint disease

- The stiff neck.
- The tentative handshake of rotator-cuff atrophy, difficulty getting in/out of sleeves.
- Stiff hips/knees.
- Kyphosis and protuberant abdomen suggestive of osteoporosis.

Self-neglect

- Dirty hands/face/body.
- Dirty clothing, evidence of incontinence.
- Unshaven, hair unkempt.
- Neglected nails.

Nutrition

- Obesity.
- Protein–energy undernutrition—compare weight with previous records. Signs of recent weight loss or extreme cachexia.
- Hydration.

Conversation

- Appropriate?
- Dyspnoea?
- Good account of circumstances?
- Plausible, with obvious lacunae?
- Mood?
- Speech—dysphasia, dysarthria, weak rapid Parkinsonian speech.
- Emotional lability.

Formal examination

- Extrasystoles—common and seldom significant.
- Neglected breast cancer.
- Displaced apex beat—due to chest deformity which also affects traditional radiation of mumurs.
- Peripheral pulses—palpate and auscultate.
- Abdomen—ribs tend to sit over pelvis, so hard to ballot kidneys, distended bladder, faecal impaction.
- Defective up-gaze—common, dubious significance.
- Ankle jerks—usually present—plantar strike often the best technique.

Pharmacological treatment: special considerations

The elderly consume most drugs (prescribed or OTC). The oldest 15% of the population receive 40% of all drug prescriptions. Older people are:
- More sensitive to drugs (weight, renal function, etc).
- More susceptible to side-effects and adverse effects.
- More likely to have side-effects that have serious sequelae.

Pharmacokinetics and pharmacodynamics

Pharmacokinetics (**what the body does to the drug**) and pharmacodynamics (**what the drug does to the body**) are **both affected by ageing**. Examples include:
- Slower gastric emptying.
- Increased ratio of adipose to lean tissue (increased volume of distribution for fat-soluble drugs, e.g. diazepam).
- Reduced plasma albumin.
- Altered liver metabolism—affects first pass (chlormethiazole and paracetamol).
- Reduced renal clearance (very important when a drug excreted by the kidney has a narrow therapeutic index, e.g. digoxin).
- Increased receptor sensitivity (psychoactive drugs and warfarin).

When problems arise there are often many causes

Example

Nellie Smith doesn't get out much because of her arthritic knees. She is prescribed an NSAID:
- Decides indigestion is normal at her age (expectations)
- Has a haematemesis (more prone to side-effects)

continued on p. 28

- Collapses (impaired homeostasis, exacerbated by her frusemide)
- Fractures her hip (co-existing osteoporosis)
- Is not found until the next day (social factors—lives alone)
- Is admitted but has complications (need for speed to avoid complications of immobility)
- Antibiotics are prescribed (iatrogenic—third generation cephalosporins should be avoided if possible)
- Develops *Clostridium difficile* diarrhoea from which she may die . . . .

Was the NSAID indicated initially?

Multiple pathology means multiple therapy

Older people on several drugs are:
- More likely to experience side-effects, drug interactions and adverse drug reactions.
- Likely to have problems with concordance, especially if confused.
- Often on a drug to treat the side-effects of another!

Reviewing the drugs—repeat prescriptions

Review your patient's problem list and prioritize the treatable. The patient is usually on many drugs already. For each drug consider:
- If the likely benefit outweighs the risk? (e.g. Mr Roland, 74 years old, is on warfarin for AF, has dementia, is prone to falls and is found to have an unexpected INR of 7.2: stop the warfarin and you may save his life.)
- Still indicated? (Oxybutinin, sulphonylurea, etc. are often continued with little evidence of efficacy.)
- 'Nicest' drug for the job? (e.g. clarithromycin has fewer gastric side-effects than erythromycin.)
- Is the drug causing the symptoms? (e.g. nausea or confusion due to codeine; frusemide and fludrocortisone are an illogical combination.)
- Could a single agent replace two? (e.g. ACE inhibitor for hypertension with CCF.)
- Is the formulation/route of administration the best? (e.g. syrups and patches may help.)
- Timings appropriate? (e.g. once-a-day or twice-a-day options aid adherence for the patient or visiting carers.)
- Aids to administration? (e.g. spacer for inhalers, no childproof tops.)
- Aids to adherence? (e.g. dosette box.)
- Regular or 'as required'? (Analgesics are usually best given on a regular basis.)
- Does the patient understand the medications and any precautions? (Supply written information and record advice in the notes.)
- Cheapest? (If there are equivalents e.g. proton pump inhibitors).

Should a new drug be started?

- With the aim of cure or disease modification, symptom control, or primary or secondary prevention.
- Start low, go slow but increase the dose until in the therapeutic range or side-effects develop.
- Give a drug for long enough before deciding it is ineffective, e.g. antidepressants.
- Where the aim is prevention, consider the overall burden of pathology and drugs, but avoid therapeutic nihilism.

How many drugs are reasonable?

Cardiac guidelines in many countries, including NICE Guidelines for treatment after MI in the UK, recommend multiple drugs:
- β-blocker
- aspirin
- ACE-inhibitor
- statin
- with heart failure—loop diuretic and spironolactone
- with diabetes—insulin in the acute phase, usual treatment later
- with AF—warfarin or aspirin and dipyridamole
- with angina—nicorandil.

Summary: the overall picture

- If there are multiple drugs, are they all essential?
- Try to avoid drugs to treat the side-effects of another drug.
- Look for potential interactions.

- If the patient has renal failure, don't rely on memory, check every drug against the list in the BNF.
- The patient will change. Always review medication. Is secondary prevention still appropriate?

Surgery in elderly patients

Obligatory versus facultative
The former category includes resection of a colonic carcinoma or fixation of a hip fracture, the latter includes life-enhancing procedures, such as elective hip replacement or cataract extraction.

Emergency versus elective
At age over 75 years, the mortality for emergency surgery is 60–80%.

The main risk factors for elective surgical patients are:

1 Cardiac: infarction during preceding 3 months or failure.

2 Respiratory: chronic obstructive lung disease, current smoking.

3 CNS: stroke during preceding 3 months, dementia.

4 Metabolic: diabetes, steroid medication, renal failure.

5 Significantly overweight or underweight.

6 Frailty and poor mobility.

Perioperative care
The amount that can be achieved pre-operatively depends on the urgency of surgery. For elective surgery, patients can be encouraged to stop smoking and improve their fitness (often not achievable if the surgery is for chronic pain, e.g. knee replacement). It may be possible to improve gross protein–energy undernutrition (by nasogastric tube if necessary) and optimize pre-existing drugs. Check whether the patient is on warfarin (replace with heparin if necessary) and whether other drugs should be given on the morning of surgery — it may be better to stop ACE inhibitors the day before. It is essential to correct heart failure, salt and water depletion, respiratory infection and severe anaemia. The skill of the anesthetist is as important as the surgeon in ensuring good operative outcome; frail old people are usually assessed pre-operatively by a senior anaesthetist who will decide whether general or regional anaesthesia is appropriate.

Ageing affects the pharmacokinetics and pharmacodynamics of many anaesthetic drugs. Pre-medicants are often avoided in the very old and reduced doses are needed for many drugs. During surgery the aim is to avoid episodes of excessive hypotension after induction of anaesthesia or large blood loss, or the combination of hypertension and tachycardia after noxious stimulation. Special care is also needed to avoid pressure damage and maintain body temperature. Post-operative analgesia requires careful control to maximize pain relief with minimal sedation or respiratory depression.

Post-operative complications
1 Respiratory infection — especially high-risk subjects resulting from atelectasis due to suppression of sighing by pain (abdominal surgery) or sedation.

2 Confusion — commonest on day 3 or 4 and following orthopaedic rather than general surgical procedures, possibly related to cerebral fat embolism. Other causes are mentioned in Chapter 4 under Acute confusional states, drugs and alcohol or their abrupt withdrawal being particularly important. Another predictable cause is hyponatraemia caused by bladder irrigation during prostatectomy. Sensory deprivation is a risk factor, as is discomfort due to pain or bladder distension.

3 Cardiac failure (in 5–10% of surgical patients over 65 years) — sometimes due to over-enthusiastic fluid replacement.

4 MI (1–4%) — half are painless — 'failure to thrive' post-operatively — comparison with a pre-operative ECG can assist the diagnosis.

5 Stroke (3% of patients over 80 years of age undergoing surgery).

6 DVT — 25–33%; it is important to follow prophylactic guidelines.

7 Pressure sores (see also Chapter 15).

Further information

Barat, I., Andreasen F., Damsgaard E.M. (2000) The consumption of drugs by 75-year-old individuals living in their own homes. *European Journal of Clinical Pharmacology* **56**, 501–9.

McMurdo, M.E. (2000) A healthy old age: realistic or futile goal? *British Medical Journal* **321**, 1149–51.

NICE website: www.nice.org.uk/nice-web

Sear, J. W. & Higham, H. (2002) Issues in the perioperative management of the elderly patient with cardiovascular disease. *Drugs & Aging* **19**(6), 429–51

Thomas, H.F., Sweetnam, P.M., Janchawee, B. & Luscombe, D.K. (1999) Polypharmacy among older men in South Wales. *European Journal of Clinical Pharmacology* **55**, 411–15.

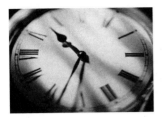

Old Age Psychiatry

Age changes

Brain weight decreases by 20% by the age of 90 years, there is selective neuronal loss of between 5% and 50% and the cells tend to shrink. There is also a 15–20% reduction in synapses in the frontal lobes. Lipofuscin accumulates in some cells, but its significance is uncertain. Plaques and tangles are found in aged brains but seldom in middle-aged ones. Granulovacuolar degeneration can often be found in the hippocampus and occasional vascular amyloid deposits are seen in cortical blood vessels. All these changes are more pronounced in Alzheimer's disease (AD).

Performance in intelligence testing, learning ability, short-term memory and reaction time tend to decline with age but often not significantly until about the age of 75 years.

Sleep

There is a positive correlation between increasing age and complaints of poor sleep. Studies indicate that sleep becomes shorter, lighter and more broken, with greater difficulty getting back to sleep again. Stages 3 and 4 of sleep are rarely attained and periods of rapid-eye-movement sleep are also infrequent. Apnoeic episodes are commoner. The worst sleep patterns are found in demented patients, who often also become much more confused in the evening or night ('sundowning'). If simple corrective measures do not help, a short course of a hypnotic may be justified.

Factors that disturb sleep patterns

- Anxiety
- Depression
- Pain
- Discomfort due to constipation
- Urgency, frequency, nocturia
- Restless legs
- Cramps
- Nocturnal cough or breathlessness
- Daytime napping
- Unrealistic expectations
- Drugs (theophylline, sympathomimetics)
- Drug withdrawal (sedatives, hypnotics)

Simple advice for poor sleepers

- Rise at a regular and early hour
- Maintain activity during the day
- Avoid coffee or tea during the evening
- Do not go to bed hungry
- Wind down before trying to get to sleep
- Take a warm milky drink in the evening
- Do not go to bed too early

Problem drinking

- Repeated ingestion leading to dependency, physical disease or other harm.
- Consumption peaks at age 55 and declines thereafter. One survey has shown that 17% of

over 60s have a problem and 12% are heavy drinkers. The usual problem is daily dosing rather than bingeing—often concealed. Older people may have particular problems with alcohol if their balance or cognition is already impaired, with obesity or malnutrition and alcohol predisposes to hypothermia.

• Treatment entails total withdrawal: delirium tremens is controlled with chlordiazepoxide.

The Institute of Alcohol Studies produces a useful fact sheet.

'Graduate drinkers'

M = F
• Falls, confusion, gastrointestinal effects, self-neglect, anxiety, depression, hallucinations, Wernicke's encephalopathy, dementia, liver and heart complications

'Late-onset drinkers'

F > M
• Attempt to assuage loneliness and sadness
• Depression common
• Complications similar to group 1

Anxiety

Anxiety is very common in older people and may accompany depression, dementia and physical illness or may cause physical symptoms (palpitations, breathlessness, giddiness, abdominal discomfort, bowel fixation). Always consider anxiety or depression in recurrent attenders in a GP or hospital setting. Treatment is by reassurance or cognitive therapy, but if severe and amounting to panic attacks, SSRIs are the drugs of choice.

Paraphrenia (persistent delusional disorder)

This is a late-life schizophreniform paranoid psychosis in which personality and affect are well preserved and there is no thought disorder.

It most often affects unmarried women who live alone, especially those who suffer from deafness. There is often a highly structured system of delusions and hallucinations, which may have a sexual content or which may relate to electrical appliances, for example. The response to antipsychotic drugs is good if concordance can be achieved. Newer agents, such as low-dose risperidone, cause fewer long-term side-effects but increase the drug bill.

Causes of hallucinations

• Paraphrenia
• Poor vision
• Bereavement
• Depression
• Acute brain syndrome (including drugs, e.g. dopaminergic treatment for Parkinson's disease)
• Dementia

Depression

Prevalence
Depression occurs in around 10–15% of people aged over 65 years and is severe in 3%. The most important thing is to consider the possibility. If you are not sure, ask the patient—most will tell you and there is a surprisingly good correlation between a yes/no answer to that question and a full psychiatric assessment. For an intermediate approach, screening tools such as the Geriatric Depression Scale (15-point version) or the BASDEC (Brief Assessment Schedule Depression Cards) may be helpful. The latter, which was developed on a medicine for the elderly ward, has the questions in large print on cards so you don't have to yell 'are you so depressed you have thought of killing yourself?' to a deaf patient on an open ward. Many old, ill people in hospital are anxious, lose their appetite, can't sleep or concentrate and so in the list of features below, physical aspects are least helpful and anhedonia, perhaps the most.

Features

- Association with physical illness. Most chronic illness is associated with depression. Growing evidence suggests that there may be a subtype of depression in later life, characterized by a distinct clinical presentation and an association with cerebrovascular disease.
- Somatization of symptoms, hypochondriasis.
- Pervasive anhedonia ('when did you last enjoy anything?').
- Guilt, worthlessness, low self-esteem.
- Hopelessness and helplessness.
- Apathy or agitation, anxiety, delusions.
- Sleep disturbance.
- Withdrawal, poor concentration and memory ('pseudodementia').
- Self-neglect, malnutrition, dehydration.
- Suicide risk.

In almost all industrialized countries, men aged 75 years and older have the highest suicide rate among all age groups. Whereas in younger age groups suicide attempts are often impulsive acts, suicide attempts in older people are often long planned and involve high-lethality methods. These characteristics, in addition to the fact that elderly are more fragile and frequently live alone, more often lead to fatal outcome. In later life, in both sexes, major depression is the most common diagnosis in those who attempt or complete suicide. A previous serious attempt, bereavement and isolation all point to high risk.

Treatment

Supportive

This involves counselling, relieving loneliness and practical measures, e.g. benefits check. Depression is often best managed with help of the local old age psychiatry service. In most areas this is a multi-professional group, with Community Psychiatric Nurses (CPNs), social workers and a consultant. The team will carry out further assessment if necessary—usually in the patient's own home and will support them to continue with medication, etc. The old age psychiatry service may run a day hospital— many have different days for clients with depression or psychosis and dementia. Other options might include referral to Cruse Bereavement Care or arranging a day centre.

Sometimes the focus is on a patient but the health needs of their carer are overlooked. Depression is extremely common amongst carers and it is essential to recognize this and offer support, such as arranging respite care or a sitting service such as Crossroads, before deterioration in the carer's mental health precipitates a crisis.

Drugs

SSRIs are the drugs of choice, having fewer sedating and anticholinergic effects than the tricyclic antidepressants and being relatively safe in overdose. Nausea, diarrhoea and restlessness can occur. To minimize nausea, start at a very low dose for the 1st week and gradually increase. Give a simple explanation of the chemical basis of depression and explain that depression can't just be shaken off by 'counting your blessings', or having a bit more moral fibre! Patients may have had bad experiences with benzodiazepines in the past and so stress that these drugs are different, that they do not usually make them feel dopey but will need to be stopped gradually when no longer needed. Explain to the patient that any nausea will wear off and strongly reinforce the need to stick with the tablets for at least 6 weeks before expecting the cloud to lift. Information sheets can be useful. Treatment should be continued for a year or possibly even for life in severe cases.

There is no clear evidence that one SSRI is more efficacious or better tolerated by elderly patients than another. Other features may influence the choice of agent. For example, fluoxetine, fluvoxamine and paroxetine are more likely to be involved in significant drug–drug interactions than citalopram or sertraline. Everyone has their own favourites but our current practice for most patients is citalopram starting with 10 mg. In special situation, the following are used: mirtazapine (a pre-synaptic α_2-antagonist which increases noradrenergic and serotinergic transmission) where appetite stimulation is needed, trazadone (tricyclic with few antimuscarinic effects) if sedation is needed and venlafaxine (a serotonin and noradrenaline re-uptake inhibitor) for resistant depression. If nausea is a major problem on SSRIs, lofepramine (a tricyclic with few antimuscarinic side effects), building from 70 mg may be helpful.

Electroconvulsive therapy

Electroconvulsive therapy (ECT) is compara-tively sure, quick and safe in severe cases but most psychiatrists are now very reluctant to consider ECT because of the bad press it has re-ceived. This is a great pity as patients who were previously 'brought back' to a useful life now sometimes linger and die on their medication.

Dementia

Dementia, of which AD is the commonest cause, is a public health problem of enormous magnitude.

What is dementia?

Dementia is a **syndrome** (lots of causes) of **ac-quired** (not learning difficulties), **chronic** (lasts months to years), **global** (not just memory or just language problems) impairment of higher brain function, in an **alert patient** (not drowsy), which **interferes with the ability to cope** with daily living (it doesn't usually matter if an old person doesn't know 'it's Tuesday' but if he or she doesn't know 'it's winter' he or she might freeze).

Remember:

My (memory)
Old (orientation)
Grandmother (grasp)
Converses (communication)
Pretty (personality change)
Badly (behaviour disorder)
(from Brice Pitt, Emeritus Professor of Old Age Psychiatry at St Mary's, London).

Dementia contrasts with **delirium**, an acute confusional state with impaired consciousness. A person can become delirious at any age, but frail older people often become confused when they are ill. An acute confusional state resolves as the underlying illness (e.g. chest or urinary in-fection) gets better. However, delirium is partic-ularly common on a background of dementia, in which case the confusion will improve but only to a limited extent.

Clinical features of acute confusion

- Onset typically abrupt
- Marked fluctuation: lucid intervals
- Altered consciousness
- Inability to sustain, focus or shift attention
- Disturbed cognition
- Delusions and hallucinations
- Fear, bewilderment, restlessness or hypoactivity
- Possibly signs of underlying cause

Causes of acute confusion

Intracranial
- Infarction—'silent'; often frontal
- Infection—meningoencephalitis
- Injury—head injury, fat embolism
- Iatrogenic—drugs acting on CNS (including abrupt withdrawal, e.g. tranquillizers)

Extracranial
- Infection—especially chest and urine
- Metabolic—fluid and electrolyte imbalance, hypoglycaemia, hypothermia
- Anoxia—cardiac or respiratory failure, 'silent' myocardial infarction, carbon monox-ide poisoning
- Toxic—alcohol, drugs
- Nutritional—Wernicke's encephalopathy

Treatment is summarized as follows:
1 Plentiful reassurance and explanation: avoid confrontation.
2 Treat underlying cause, correct fluid and electrolyte imbalance, correct nutritional deficiencies.
3 Environmental—use a dim light overnight.
4 Restlessness, agitation: haloperidol (cheap) risperidone (better side-effect profile but more

expensive) or if neuroleptics are to be avoided try chlormethiazole or lorazepam.

Causes of the dementia syndrome

The **primary dementias**, where the disease mainly affects the neurons in the brain, include AD, Lewy body disease, other frontotemporal lobar atrophies including Pick's disease and frontotemporal dementia and Creutzfeldt—Jakob disease.

The commonest **secondary dementia**, in which the neuronal damage is secondary to pathology in other tissues, is vascular dementia (which includes multiple small infarcts and white matter ischaemia). CADASIL (see below) is a familial microangiopathy that usually presents in middle age with recurrent TIAs or stroke. The mean age of onset for TIAs and/or stroke is 45 years, but the range extends from the early 20s to the 60s. Other important causes are drugs and alcohol, endocrine and metabolic problems such as thyroid dysfunction, recurrent or severe hypoglycaemia, post-hypoxia, nutritional problems such as vitamin B_{12} deficiency, brain tumours, trauma and infections including syphilis and HIV.

Remember:

Drugs and alcohol
Eyes and ears
Metabolic
Emotional (really, psychiatric problems)
Nutritional
Trauma and tumours
Infections
Atheroma—vascular dementia.

How common is dementia?

Dementia is rare below the age of 55 years but the prevalence of dementia increases dramatically with age to about **3% in the over 65s** and rising to about **20% in the over 80s**. There is a slight female preponderance. In elderly people, AD probably accounts for half to two-thirds of cases of dementia. About 700 000 people in England and Wales have dementia.

What happens in dementia?

The onset of dementia is insidious with gradual changes in memory and concentration, thinking processes, language use, personality, behaviour and orientation. Short-term memory is impaired early—long-term recall is often much better. Thinking becomes rigid and concrete. The condition progresses to obvious problems with short-term memory and managing basic activities of daily living, increasing disorientation and sometimes difficult or distressing behaviour such as night-time wandering, aggression or apathy. A tendency to lose things easily turns into paranoia and even delusions. Constant repetition of the same questions can be very trying for carers. Eventually, the patient is completely disorientated, no longer recognizes close family members, ceases to communicate and becomes doubly incontinent, bed-bound and totally dependent. Sadly survival is often 8–10 years.

Why does dementia matter?

Dementia is a devastating condition for the **patient,** while insight is preserved, and their **family** who witness the progressive deterioration. For the spouse this has been likened to 'being bereaved without being widowed'. Dementia also has major **economic** consequences. Demographic changes are resulting in marked increases in the oldest old, one in five of whom may have dementia, a major cause of dependency and institutional care. Politicians and **society** are beginning to grapple with the issues and the cost of providing health and social care for patients with AD. In England, the direct costs of AD have been estimated at between £7.06 billion and £14.93 billion (2001), greater than the costs of stroke, heart disease and cancer. In addition to the considerable **morbidity**, it is believed that AD is the fourth leading cause of **death** in the West. However, 'bronchopneumonia' usually appears on the death certificate. Despite this burden, dementia is only just beginning to command the attention it deserves.

How is a diagnosis of dementia made?

The **GP** is usually the first port of call, but a survey performed by the Alzheimer's Disease Society suggests that there is often difficulty in obtaining a diagnosis. Many old people are slightly forgetful and it can be difficult to distinguish ageing changes from early dementia. The term **age-associated memory impairment** is applied to a subjective complaint of forgetfulness in those over 50 years of age, with a performance on memory testing one standard deviation below the normal for a young adult. Almost 20% of people over 50 years of age meet these criteria and the significance is uncertain.

GPs may be reluctant to diagnose an 'untreatable' condition. If the patient lives alone there may be no one to give a history and unless a simple test of cognition is performed, it is easy to be misled by 'a good social front'. Suitable quick screening tests include Hodkinson's Abbreviated Mental Test Score. However, if there are family members and they are concerned there is usually a problem, whereas if only the patient is complaining the diagnosis is often anxiety, depression or 'worried well'. Although dementia may have been developing for months, the patient often presents acutely because of a social crisis (e.g. death of caring spouse) or physical crisis (any illness, often a chest or urine infection, which worsens the confusion).

Having identified possible dementia, the GP may manage the patient or **refer** to a geriatrician, an old age psychiatrist, a neurologist, or in some areas, a specialist memory clinic.

What are the aims of a clinical assessment?

Is it dementia?

A full history, with more detailed cognitive function testing, including assessment of language, visuospatial skills and reasoning (e.g. Mini-Mental State Examination (see Appendix 4), Alzheimer's Disease Assessment Scale) usually answers this question. At this stage, other conditions must be ruled out.

The **differential diagnosis** includes an acute confusional state, depression, communication difficulties due to deafness, poor vision, or language deficits, PD, schizophrenia and mania.

What type of dementia is it?

The next step is to identify the cause. The dementia may be reversible (e.g. hypothyroidism), treatment may slow disease progression (e.g. treating hypertension in vascular dementia), specific treatment may be available (e.g. AD), genetic counselling may be required (e.g. familial AD) or it may be important to avoid certain medication (e.g. neuroleptics in Lewy body disease).

There is no diagnostic test for most of the primary dementias until a post-mortem examination, so the *likely* cause is determined by the **clinical features** and the results of **investigations.** Common conditions such as vascular dementia and AD may co-exist.

Progressive deterioration is common in AD whereas step-wise deterioration is characteristic of vascular dementia. Neuropsychiatric phenomena such as delusions and hallucinations and extreme sensitivity to major tranquillizers are a feature of Lewy body disease. Parkinsonian features on examination would suggest vascular dementia or Lewy body disease. Most patients with dementia show some fluctuation, known as 'sundowning' because the confusion worsens in the evening, but this can be surprisingly marked in Lewy body disease, even affecting conscious level. Weighted scores, such as the Hachinski ischaemia score, may improve diagnostic accuracy and work is in progress to determine whether patterns of change found on neuropsychological and language testing add to diagnosis.

Investigations typically include blood tests to exclude reversible causes or other major pathology (blood count, biochemical profile, ESR, thyroid function, B_{12} and folate and syphilis serology) CXR and ECG and a CT scan or MRI. In the late stages, a CT scan usually shows cerebral atrophy but many patients with AD have a normal looking scan initially. The main purpose of the scan is to rule out a space-occupying lesion and identify major vascular disease. Genetic tests, such as determining the apolipoprotein E alleles that predispose to AD, are not routine.

Management

Management depends on the severity of the dementia, whether the patient lives alone and comprises a multi-disciplinary, multi-agency package of care. The package needs to be well co-ordinated and to evolve as the needs of the patient and carer change. Options include:

• Coping strategies and psychological techniques, reminiscence work and validation therapy.
• Optimize hearing, vision and improve general health.
• Treat other conditions which may impair cognition (e.g. anaemia, heart failure).
• Treat risk factors (e.g. hypertension in vascular dementia).
• Treat specific symptoms and behaviours (major tranquillizers, unfortunately, are often the only option).
• Education and support for carers (Alzheimer's Disease Society, Carers' National Association).
• Genetic counselling (only in rare early-onset dementias).
• Legal advice (e.g. an Enduring Power of Attorney may obviate the need for the Court of Protection at a later date, advice about driving, advance directives, etc).
• Therapy assessments (occupational therapy, speech and language therapy (for swallowing and communication) and physiotherapy; the aim is usually assessment to plan appropriate care and advise carers, rather than treat the patient).
• Assessment by social services (financial entitlements, especially attendance allowance, provision of services like home help and access to 'care management', the process by which frail old people are assessed for substantial packages of care at home or residential care).
• Regular district nurse/community psychiatric nurse support.
• Sitting services (Crossroads), day hospitals, respite care.
• Proper provision of long-term care.
This list demonstrates just how much can be done in dementia. Until recently, no specific treatment was available. Drug management focused on the effects of the disease (e.g. major tranquillizers for disturbed behaviour) but advances in our understanding of the pathological processes in AD have led to the development of drugs to ameliorate the underlying biochemical changes.

Notes on Alzheimer's disease

AD is divided into early-onset familial AD (EOFAD) and the usually sporadic late-onset form (LOAD). The pathology of both is identical with characteristic amyloid-containing extracellular **plaques** and the abnormal material which develops inside the neurons, the **neurofibrillary tangles**. It has been more than 10 years since it was first proposed that the neuronal degeneration in AD may be caused by deposition of amyloid beta-peptide (Aβ) in plaques in brain tissue. According to the amyloid hypothesis, accumulation of Aβ in the brain drives the pathogenesis of AD. The rest of the disease process, including formation of neurofibrillary tangles containing tau protein, is proposed to result from an imbalance between Aβ production and Aβ clearance.

Three genes have been linked with EOFAD and all probably increase the brain levels of the amyloid precursor protein (see Table 4.1).

Risk factors for Alzheimer's disease

• Down's syndrome. Essentially all people with trisomy 21 develop the neuropathological hallmarks of AD after 40 years of age. More than half such individuals also show clinical evidence of cognitive decline. The presumed reason is the lifelong over-expression of the amyloid precursor protein and resultant over production of the Aβ-amyloid.
• Age.
• Female sex.
• Apolipoprotein E4 genotype.
• Head injury.
• Elevated homocysteine levels (can be decreased by folate*).

GENES AND ALZHEIMER'S DISEASE

		Chromosome	
EOFAD			
β-amyloid	APP	21	Associated with Down's syndrome
Presenilin 1	PSEN1	14q	Commonest gene defect in EOFAD
Presenilin 2	PSEN'	1q	
LOAD			
Apolipoprotein E	ApoE	19q	Polymorphic: e2 e3 e4 are the common isoforms. e4 is associated with atherosclerosis, coronary heart disease, vascular dementia, early and late onset AD
?		10, 12	At least four other loci are postulated

EOFAD, early-onset familial Alzheimer's disease; LOAD, late-onset Alzheimer's disease.

Table 4.1 Genes associated with familial and sporadic AD.

Protective factors for Alzheimer's disease

- Education (partly a threshold effect, but ? confounding with other associations with social class, e.g. diet high in antioxidants*).
- Continued brain activity (keep reading!).
- Tobacco (may be the nicotinic effect on cholinergic transmission, but not worth it).
- Wine and coffee (so it's not all bad news!).
- Exercise.
- Diet rich in foods containing vitamin E but not vitamin E supplements*.
- Non-steroidal anti-inflammatory drugs and aspirin.
- Hormone replacement therapy (observational data but as hormone replacement therapy users are fitter than average, trials are needed).
- Treatment with a statin (could be reduction in vascular damage but trials are needed).

The metabolism of acetylcholine
(see Fig. 4.1)

Cholinergic transmission could be enhanced by increasing the availability of the precursor, via direct stimulation of the receptors or by preventing the breakdown of endogenous acetylcholine. Three drugs, which are all acetylcholinesterase inhibitors, are available (Table 4.2). Acetylcholinesterase inhibitors are widely available in some countries but in the

UK should be prescribed according to NICE guidelines (2001):
- Diagnosis of AD made in a specialist clinic.
- MMSE ≥ 12.
- Carer's views considered and feasible to expect compliance.
- Drug continued if cognitive or behavioural benefit (stable MMSE indicates benefit as decline is expected).
- Six-monthly review and drug stopped if benefit no longer apparent or MMSE falls below 12.

*Large trials are in progress with vitamins B_6, B_{12}, C, β-carotene and folic acid, oestrogens, celecoxib, simvastatin, selenium and ginkgo and will report between 2003 and 2008. Other options include β- and γ-secretase inhibitors (to modulate amyloid plaque formation) or vaccination with Aβ following successful studies in a mouse model of AD. However, the specific treatments for AD which are currently in use are based on earlier work showing that the neurons which bear the brunt of the damage are those which use acetylcholine to transmit messages.

ALZHEIMER'S DISEASE—CHOLINESTERASE INHIBITORS

Drug name	Recommended dose	Common side-effects	Possible drug interactions
Galantamine Prevents the breakdown of acetylcholine and stimulates nicotinic receptors to release more acetylcholine in the brain	4 mg, twice a day Increase after 4 weeks to 8 mg twice a day After another 4 weeks, increase to 12 mg twice a day if well tolerated	Nausea, vomiting, diarrhoea, weight loss	Prescription with inhibitors of cytochrome P450, e.g. paroxetine, amitriptyline or ketoconazole may cause cholinergic toxicity due to decreased metabolism of galantamine. Caution with all three drugs in sick sinus syndrome, peptic ulcer and hence NSAIDs, COPD, urine retention
Rivastigmine Prevents the breakdown of acetylcholine and butyrylcholine (a brain chemical similar to acetylcholine) in the brain	1.5 mg, twice a day Increase by 3 mg/day every 2 weeks to 6 mg twice a day Continue up to 6 mg twice a day if well tolerated	Nausea, vomiting, weight loss, upset stomach, muscle weakness	
Donepezil Prevents the breakdown of acetylcholine in the brain	5 mg, once a day (nocte to minimize nausea) Increase after 4–6 weeks to 10 mg once a day	Nausea, diarrhoea, vomiting	

Table 4.2

Although the licensed indication is AD, trials have shown benefit in Lewy body dementia and vascular dementia, and so the lack of diagnostic precision is not a danger.

Although the cholinergic system is primarily affected other neurotransmitter systems are involved and memantine, an N-methyl-D-aspartate receptor antagonist (which reduces glutamate-induced neurotoxicity) has just been licensed in the UK for the treatment of moderate to severe AD. The fact that it may also be useful in vascular dementia, neuropathic pain and glaucoma indicates that this is a rather non-specific approach.

Frontotemporal dementia

Frontotemporal dementia is characterized by gradual changes in personality, social behavior, and language ability. Symptoms depend on whether the damage has primarily affected the right (behavioral problems) or left side (language deficits) of the frontal and anterior temporal lobes that control executive functioning. Frontotemporal dementia usually develops between 35 and 75 years of age and so, although it is rare (about 3% of dementia cases), it may present at an age when patients are labelled with AD. Orientation and memory are better preserved than in AD.

Pathologically, it is characterized by neurofibrillary tangles. These are known to be abnormally processed microtubule proteins. The microtubule-associated protein tau promotes tubulin polymerization and has a role in stabilizing the microtubules that are responsible for neuronal architecture and transport. A mu-

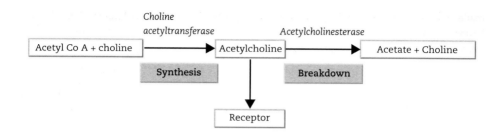

Fig. 4.1 The metabolism of acetylcholine.

tation in the *tau* gene causes a form of frontotemporal dementia called frontotemporal dementia with Parkinsonism linked to chromosome 17 (FTDP-17). Mutations in the *tau* gene impair the binding of tau protein to the microtubule and so frontotemporal dementia is one of the 'tauopathies'.

CADASIL

Cerebral autosomal dominant arteriopathy with subcortical infarcts and leukoencephalopathy is characterized by a history of migraine, mid-adult (30s–60s) onset of cerebrovascular disease progressing to dementia, and diffuse white matter lesions and subcortical infarcts on neuroimaging. The pathological hallmark of CADASIL is electron dense granules in the media of arterioles that can often be identified by electron microscopic evaluation of skin biopsies. More than 90% of patients have mutations in the *Notch3* gene (chromosomal locus 19p). Molecular genetic testing is available.

Transient global amnesia

A curious episodic disorder predominantly affecting older people. It is of unknown cause and is not predictive of stroke or dementia. In an episode the person remains alert and capable of high-level intellectual activity (e.g. driving), but if questioned may be perplexed and has impaired memory for past and present events.

Features
• Sudden-onset amnesia—retrograde for recent events, anterograde preventing new memories being laid down.
• Bemusement, perplexity, disorientation, repetitive questioning.
• Preservation of alertness, verbal fluency, motor activity.
• Duration a few hours, although complete recovery may take a few days; low recurrence rate.

Self-neglect

Old people are not infrequently encountered living in conditions of extreme degradation with total disregard for hygiene and self-care, the 'senile squalor syndrome'. Some will be found to have mental illness but others appear normal despite hoarding vast quantities of rubbish. This has been termed the Diogenes syndrome after Diogenes of Sinope, the ancient Greek philosopher who showed his contempt for material things by living in a barrel. He believed that happiness is attained by satisfying one's natural needs in the cheapest and easiest ways possible. In this context, the perpetrator is seen to have

Risk factors associated with self-neglect

• Dementia.
• Depression.
• Bereavement and isolation.
• Disability.
• Alcohol.
• Previous psychiatric disorder.
• Mental subnormality.
• Obsessive-compulsive disorder.
• Lifelong difficult personality/eccentricity.

made a bizarre lifestyle choice, rather than having an illness, but the condition may lead to hypothermia, malnutrition and infections as well as vigorous protests from the neighbours!

Further information

Adshead, F., Cody, D.D. & Pitt, B. (1992) BASDEC: a novel screening instrument for depression in the elderly. *British Medical Journal* **305**, 397.

Alcohol and the Elderly: ias fact sheet. www.ias.org.uk/factsheets/alcoholelderly.pdf

Alzheimer's Disease Education and Referral (ADEAR) Centre's National Institute of Aging website: http://www.alzheimers.org/

Alzheimer's Disease Society's website: http://www.alzheimers.org.uk/

Medical Clinics of North America 2002 May, **86**(3). This volume of the *Medical Clinics of North America* is devoted to different aspects of dementia.

Dominguez, D.I. & De Strooper, B. (2002) Novel therapeutic strategies provide the real test for the amyloid hypothesis of Alzheimer's disease. *Trends in Pharmacolgical Science* **23**(7), 324–30.

Hardy, J. & Selkoe, D.J. (2002) Amyloid hypothesis of Alzheimer's disease: progress and problems on the road to therapeutics. *Science* **297**(5580), 353–61.

Lindsay, J., Laurin, D., Verreault, R. *et al.* (2002) Risk factors for Alzheimer's disease: a prospective analysis from the Canadian Study of Health and Aging. *American Journal of Epidemiology*, **156**(5), 445–53.

Lowin, A., Knapp, M. & McCrone, P. (2001) Alzheimer's disease in the UK: comparative evidence on cost of illness and volume of health services research funding. *International Journal of Geriatric Psychiatry* **16**(12), 1143–8.

McKeith, I.G., Burn, D.J., Ballard, C.G. *et al.* (2003) Dementia with Lewy bodies. *Seminars in Clinical Neuropsychiatry* **8**, 46–57.

NICE guidelines for prescription of Alzheimer's disease drugs (2001): Alzheimer's disease—donepezil, rivastigmine and galantamine. Technology appraisal number 19. http://www.nice.org.uk/Cat.asp?c=14400

Rosenberg, R.N. (2000) The molecular and genetic basis of Alzheimer's disease: the end of the beginning: the 2000 Wartenberg lecture. *Neurology* **54**(11), 2045–54.

Szanto, K., Gildengers, A., Mulsant, B.H., Brown, G., Alexopoulos, G.S. & Reynolds, C.F. IIIrd (2002) Identification of suicidal ideation and prevention of suicidal behaviour in the elderly. *Drugs & Aging* **19**(1), 11–24.

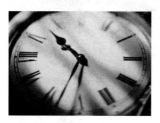

Falls and Immobility

Falls

Introduction
- Falls are *common*: one-third of over 65 year olds and one-half of over 80 year olds living in the community fall per year; and 50% of these are multiple falls.
- Women fall more often than men do.
- Older people in *nursing homes* fall most often of all, because of their increasing frailty.
- Falls are *multi-factorial*, i.e. caused by the interplay between internal and external risk factors.
- Falls are not an inevitable part of ageing.
- Falls have important *sequelae*.

Causes of falls
Most falls arise as a combination of internal factors, including gait and balance problems, medical, psychiatric and drug-related causes, and external causes, usually environmental.

A simple mnemonic for falls

DAME (reminds you that they are most common in women):
Drugs (don't forget alcohol)
Age-related changes (gait, sensory impairment)
Medical (cardiovascular disease, heart disease, Parkinson's disease (PD))
Environmental (obstacles, lighting, etc.).

Internal risk factors
Effects of ageing
- Body sway increases with age.
- Women have more body sway them men at any age.
- Reaction time slows down.
- Reflexes may be reduced.
- Walking patterns become less efficient and more irregular — will be made worse by unsuitable footwear and neurological disease.

Medical causes of falls
1 *Impaired sensory input*
  (a) Visual impairment (cataracts, glaucoma and inappropriate or dirty glasses) makes detection of hazards difficult and dark adaption is much slower, increasing the risk of falls at night.
  (b) Impaired hearing and balance including vertigo and dizziness.
  (c) Peripheral neuropathy makes walking difficult and potentially dangerous.
2 *Drug-related*
  (a) Sedatives such as benzodiazepines and opiates impair insight and balance.
  (b) Postural hypotension is often iatrogenic, e.g. diuretics for dependent oedema, treatment of PD.
  (c) Cardiac arrhythmias may be iatrogenic, e.g. secondary to tricyclic antidepressants.
  (d) Extrapyramidal side-effects secondary to neuroleptic medications.
  (e) Polypharmacy, i.e. being on four or more medications correlates strongly with the risk of falling.
  (f) Excess alcohol.
3 *Gait abnormalities*
  (a) PD: the patient has difficulty getting going,

the gait is shuffling and there is retropulsion.

(b) Hemiplegic gait: steps are slower, shorter and the gait is less smooth because the affected leg swings out in an arc.

(c) Cerebellar disease: a wide-base unsteady gait.

(d) Sensory ataxia: patient obviously watching the ground and their feet rather than looking ahead.

(e) Normal pressure hydrocephalus: again a wide-base ataxic gait.

(f) Antalgic gait: asymmetrical because the patient puts their weight on the side with the painful joint for as short a time as possible.

(g) Proximal myopathy: secondary to steroids and osteomalacia for example produces a waddling gait.

(h) 'Scissoring' gait: osteoarthritis of the hips severely reduces the range of flexion at the pelvis during walking.

(i) Foot drop: high-stepping, foot slapping gait, e.g. a common peroneal nerve palsy secondary to a plaster cast fitting too tightly.

4 *Reduced cerebral perfusion*

(a) Cardiac—rate and rhythm changes and inability to maintain steady BP (see Chapter 9).

(b) Cerebrovascular transient brain-stem ischaemia (see Chapter 7).

(c) Syncope: carotid sinus hypersensitivity, aortic stenosis (see Chapter 9) or situational syncope, secondary to cough, micturition, etc.

5 *Epilepsy*

The history is suggestive if there was a prodrome, e.g. smell of burning in temporal lobe epilepsy, longer duration of LOC with tonic clonic movements and cyanosis, incontinence and slow recovery associated with confusion and drowsiness (see Chapter 8).

6 *Dizziness and unsteadiness*

These are all descriptions of vague (heart-sink) symptoms. There are many possible causes, but they can be simplified into:

(a) Vascular disease which may respond to aspirin.

(b) Clinical cervical spondylosis, which may improve if a neck collar is worn.

(c) Review and stop any implicated medications including diuretics and advise to reduce alcohol intake if appropriate.

7 *Psychiatric problems*

(a) Dementia, especially Lewy body dementia.

(b) Delirium.

(c) Depression.

(d) Psychiatric medications, including antipsychotic medications and antidepressants.

External risk factors

• Older people tend to live in older housing, which may need repairs.

• Poor lighting, especially near stairs.

• A lifetime's clutter.

• Inappropriate footwear, slippers are well named.

• Incorrect use of walking aids.

• Pets underfoot.

• Trailing electrical cables.

• Unfamiliar environment, e.g. hospital or a care home.

Sequelae of falls

1 *Physical injuries*: occur in about one-half of reported falls.

• Soft-tissue bruising may require analgesics if mobility is to be maintained. Trauma may be reflected in raised muscle-enzyme levels.

• Breaks in skin may be very slow to heal and grafting may be required.

• Fractures: orthopaedic treatment may be required in about 6% of falls.

• Friction burns from synthetic carpet when attempting to get up.

• Falls on to a fire or a hot surface, e.g. radiator, may result in a burn.

• Central-cord lesion leading to quadriplegia in patients with spinal cord compromised by spondylosis.

2 *Psychological injury:*

• Fear of falling is increasingly being recognised as a common and important consequence of falls with significant effects on the future well-being of older people.

• Loss of confidence and mobility may result in older people becoming housebound or in need of residential care.

- Anxiety/depression about the future.
3 *Social injury:*
- Because of intolerable anxiety in carers (formal and informal).
- Increased demands on carer may cause antagonism.
- Need to move to safer surroundings may separate faller from current supporters.
4 *Death:*
- As a direct consequence of the fall.
- Up to 25% of frequent fallers are dead within 1 year of presentation, not directly due to injuries but because of underlying cause of falls.

Sequelae of a long lie

(i.e. remaining on the floor for 1 h or more after falling)
- Pressure sores (see Chapter 15)
- Hypothermia may result if fall occurs in the cold, e.g. outside or in an unheated room (see Chapter 12)
- Hypostatic pneumonia
- Fifty per cent of those who lie on the floor for 1 h or more are dead within 6 months, even if no injury was sustained from the fall

---

Investigation of falls

It is essential to get a witness report of the event surrounding the fall/s because:
- The patient may play down the event for fear of consequences
- The patient may not remember blacking out, especially if the event was transitory.
- The witness can give information about the length of time of a blackout and whether there was associated tonic–clonic movements, etc.
- The patient may have cognitive impairment.
- Research shows that even cognitively intact older people living in the community do not remember the falls after 3 months.

Examination

Must be complete and thorough but pay particular attention to the following.
  the pulse rate and rhythm; massage the
    vith ECG monitoring. See Chap-
    iod and contraindications.

- Measure the BP—lying and after standing for 3 min. The drop is significant if it is more than 10 mmHg diastolic or 20 mmHg systolic and accompanied by symptoms. See Chapter 9.
- Look for sources of emboli—listen for murmurs, carotid bruits.
- Assess the CNS and look for lateralizing signs.
- Is there evidence of PD?
- Does the patient have myxoedema?
- Is there evidence of a peripheral neuropathy?
- Proximal myopathy: does the patient have difficulty getting out of the chair?
- Assess vision and hearing.
- Examine the neck movements. Does this cause dizziness?
- If the patient describes true vertigo, do the Hallpike manoevre.
- Assess the Mental Test Score.

Baseline tests
- FBC.
- TSH.
- ECG.

Further investigations

The majority of falls are caused by problems with gait and balance. If falls continue and remain unexplained then it may be appropriate to investigate more aggressively:
- Holter monitor may show evidence of arrhythmia (the current thinking is that 48-h tapes have a greater yield than 24-h tapes but there is no additional benefit from longer than this).
- Echocardiography will reveal aortic stenosis.
- Tilt table: measuring beat-to-beat variation in pulse and BP with the patient tilted to 70°. See Chapter 9 for further discussion. CT scan if multi-infarct disease suspected.
- If fits are the suspected cause, EEG, CT scan in selected cases.

Treatment

The best way of approaching the management of falls is from a multi-disciplinary and multi-agency angle. Many hospitals now offer a Falls Prevention Clinic.

- Identify and treat **all** contributing causes and risk factors.
- Refer for physiotherapy. The aims are:
  (a) Correct prescription and use of walking aids. For example, people with PD often do better with wheeled frames to avoid the disruption to the flow of movements caused by having to lift the frame up.
  (b) Improve gait pattern, e.g. encourage people with PD to take longer steps.
  (c) Teach the patient how to get up from the floor.
The current evidence shows that individually tailored exercise plans do prevent future falls.
- Refer for occupational therapy assessment to identify and remove environmental hazards and provide equipment to facilitate mobility at home, and consider moving downstairs or getting a stair-lift.
- Challenge the need for all medication. Stop those that are unnecessary and try more patient-friendly alternatives where possible.
- Give advice on appropriate footwear: low heel for good heel strike but the soles should not be so thick that sensation is lost.
  If no obvious causes are found, reduce the risks arising from the falls:
- Think about prevention of osteoporosis with calcium and vitamin D or bisphosphonates.

Falls in hospital

- Are very common
- Are associated with cognitive impairment and acute delirium
- May be due to unfamiliar surroundings and be exacerbated by disturbed sleep and change in daily routines
- May result in soft-tissue injuries and fractures
- Prevention is under-researched

- Consider the use of hip protectors.
- Maintain a constant environmental temperature.
- Soften floor coverings, i.e. carpet rooms.
- Remove obstacles and dangers, e.g. guard fire.
- Place emergency bedding where it can be reached from the floor.
- Arrange for a personally worn alarm system or for frequent visitors.
- Teach the patient how to get up from the floor without help.
- Educate the patient and their relatives about safety in the home and the risk of falls: RoSPA (Royal Society for the Prevention of Accidents) and Age Concern produce very helpful leaflets.

Hip protectors

- These are pads made from the same material as motorcycle helmets and work by diffusing the impact of a fall away from the neck of femur.
- They are worn over the greater trochanter and are incorporated in tight-fitting underpants
- Community dwelling patients need to have good standing balance so that they can get the pants on and off
- They may cause incontinence
- They tend to be well-tolerated in homes where residents are toileted regularly or wear pads
- They have been shown to be cost-effective when used in the right population

Immobility

There are degrees of reduced mobility, ranging from not being able to drive, to being housebound and to being wheelchair-dependent. Immobility increases with increasing age. Over half of over 75 year olds have difficulty getting around their own homes. Among the ambulant aged 80 years and over at least 25% will need some mechanical support when walking, such as a stick or frame. Generally, walking speed is reduced, with shorter, broader-based gait and increased time spent in 'double support', i.e. both feet in contact with the floor. Twenty per cent are totally housebound. Many older people find it difficult to climb on to a bus and if they do manage it, there are other pitfalls: getting up off the seat, walking down the crowded aisle possibly whilst the bus is still in motion and getting

IMMOBILITY CAUSED BY PAIN/STIFFNESS

In joints	In muscles	In bones
Osteoarthritis	Myositis	Osteoporosis
Rheumatoid arthritis	Polymyalgia rheumatica	Osteomalacia
Gout	Myxoedema	Paget's disease
Pseudogout	PD	Malignant disease
Infection		

Table 5.1

IMMOBILITY CAUSED BY WEAKNESS

Neuronal damage	Muscle damage	Reduced effort tolerance
Hemiplegia	Disuse	Dyspnoea
Peripheral neuropathy	Myopathy	Anaemia
Motor-neuron disease	Amyotrophy	Reduced cardiac output
Paraplegia	Hypokalaemia	

Table 5.2

PSYCHOLOGICAL CAUSES OF IMMOBILITY

Fear and anxiety	Re. falling
Manipulative behaviour	Attention seeking
Depression	Apathy reduces initiative
Dementia	Reduces insight into need to maintain mobility

Table 5.3

off at the correct stop. This coincides with the time that people are no longer able to drive because of failing vision, syncope, etc. (see Chapter 16).

Reasons for immobility

1 Pain and stiffness in bones, joints and muscles (Table 5.1). This is the most common reason.
2 Weakness, e.g. neurological or endocrine (see Table 5.2), but also generalized systemic disease.
3 Visual impairment and blindness.
4 Breathlessness secondary to pulmonary and cardiac disease.
5 Psychological problems: fear/anxiety/depression/dementia (see Table 5.3).
6 Frequent falls and fear of falling.
7 Iatrogenic, e.g. sedation, surgery (amputations and unsuccessful orthopaedic procedures).
8 Foot-care disorders, e.g. bunions and nail neglect; also severe ischaemia and infection.

Complications of immobility

Physical
- Muscle wasting (see Chapter 6)
- Osteoporosis (see Chapter 6)
- Muscle contractures
- Pressure sores (see Chapter 15)
- Hypothermia (see Chapter 12)
- Hypostatic pneumonia
- Constipation
- Incontinence
- DVT (see Chapter 9)

Psychological
- Depression
- Loss of confidence

Social
- Isolation
- Risk of institutionalization

Further information

Age Concern website: www.ageconcern.org.uk

Home and Leisure Accident Research (1988) *Accidents and Elderly People*. Department of Trade and Industry, London.

Lord, S.R., Sherrington, C. & Menz, H.B. (2001) *Falls in Older People: Risk Factors and Strategies for Prevention*. Cambridge University Press, Cambridge.

Royal Society for the Prevention of Accidents website: www.rospa.co.uk

Studenski, S. (1996) *Clinics in Geriatric Medicine — Gait and Balance Disorders*. W.B. Saunders, Philadelphia.

Wynne-Horley, D. (1991) *Living Dangerously: Risk Taking, Safety and Older People*. Centre for Policy on Ageing, London.

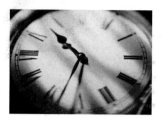

Bones, Muscles and Joints

Bones

Ageing changes

Bone structure changes throughout life owing to ongoing bone resorption by osteoclasts and bone growth by osteoblasts. With increasing age, the balance is lost leading to increased bone resorption. This in turn leads to gradual and progressive loss of bone from the age of 35 onwards. This process affects trabecular bone more than cortical bone. The bone is histologically normal but the total bone mass is markedly reduced.

Bone loss per year is 0.2% of the total from the age of 35 and this increases to 1% after the menopause in women. This means that by the age of 80, a woman will have lost 30% of her bone mass whilst a man of the same age will have lost 10%.

The shape of long bones changes with increasing age; the internal cavity increases in diameter, the outer cortical layer becomes thinner and the total bone diameter becomes expanded. These changes result in weaker bones.

Osteoporosis
Risk factors for osteoporosis
• Longevity.
• Female sex.
• Failure to maximise bone density in adolescence and early adulthood because of poor nutrition or oestrogen deficits, e.g. secondary to anorexia nervosa.

• Hormonal changes at the menopause, the fall in oestrogen causes acceleration of bone loss.
• Poor calcium intake.
• Poor calcium absorption.
• Low body weight.
• Physical inactivity.
• Drugs especially steroids, caffeine, alcohol and cigarettes.
• Maternal history of hip fracture.
• Endocrine disorders, e.g. thyrotoxicosis, Cushing's disease, hyperparathyroidism, hypopituitism.

Osteoporosis in men

• Affects 20% of men over 70 years of age
• Commonest causes are:
  (a) Hypogonadotrophic hypogonadism
  (b) Steroids
  (c) Alcohol
  (d) Hyperparathyroidism secondary to calcium malabsorption

Clinical features
Osteoporosis is asymptomatic until there has been a fracture:
• Often the first presentation is a Colles' wrist fracture in women aged 50–65 years old.
• Vertebral fractures may present as severe mid-thoracic or low back pain often with no history of trauma.
• Loss of height and dorsal kyphosis secondary to multiple vertebral fractures.

- Hip fractures: rising incidence with increasing age. Incidence rising faster than expected from demographic changes. There are now 57 000 cases per annum in the UK — 75% of which are aged over 75.
- Other fractures associated with osteoporosis include neck of humerus, pelvis and distal tibia ± fibula.

Fractured neck of femur

- Increasingly common in the ageing population
- The worldwide prediction for the number in 2050 is 6.26 million
- Presents as pain in the hip with inability to weight bear, although if it is an impacted fracture the patient may be able to walk
- The affected leg is shortened, and the hip is flexed and externally rotated
- The fracture is fixed according to its site
- The timing of the operation is controversial. The best compromise is as soon as reasonably possible when patient's medical condition is optimized
- Early mobilization
- The reasons for the fall should be sought and treated if possible
- Consider the need for treatment of osteoporosis

Fractured pelvis

- Usually the pubic rami
- Often caused by trivial trauma
- Produces pain in the groin which is worse on walking and getting up from sitting
- Treatment is conservative with analgesia and early mobilization
- Most heal within 6–8 weeks

Investigations

1 *Bone density.* The dual energy X-ray absorptiometry (DEXA) scanner measures bone density usually at the proximal femur but also of the lumbar vertebrae and calcaneum. Osteoporosis is defined as a bone mineral density (BMD) of greater than 2.5 standard deviations below that of a normal pre-menopausal woman and is expressed as a T score (i.e. T = < −2.5 SD).

2 *Ultrasound of the calcaneum* has the advantage of being cheap and portable so that it can be used in the primary care setting but has not been fully validated.

3 *Excluding causes of secondary osteoporosis:*
   (a) Serum calcium to exclude primary hyperparathyroidism.
   (b) TSH: to exclude thyrotoxicosis.
   (c) Testosterone: in men with suspected hypogonadotrophic hypogondism.
   (d) ESR, immunoglobulins to exclude myeloma.
   (e) Dexamethasone suppression test.

Complications of osteoporosis
- Fractures, as above.
- Mortality: 20% of patients who have fractured their hip are dead within 6 months of the event.
- Deformity: kyphosis, loss of height, abdominal protrusion. Cord compression is very uncommon.
- Loss of independence and risk of being admitted to a care home.
- Use of resources: 25% of UK orthopaedic beds are occupied by patients with fractured hips. The average cost is £12 000 per patient. Fractures in osteoporotic bones now account for over 1 million bed-days annually in the NHS. The cost of treatment of these patients is now more than £5 million per week.

Prevention
- Adequate nutrition.
- Calcium and vitamin D.
- Hormone replacement therapy is most useful in women in early menopause.
- Exercise: should be regular and weight-bearing, e.g. walking.
- Prophylactic use of bisphosphonates: if treatment with steroids, dose greater than 7.5 mg of prednisolone, is intended for more than 6 months.

Treatments

1 Calcium and vitamin D. It has been shown that treatment with calcium and vitamin D prevents hip fractures in older people living in care homes. Probably sufficient in the older, frailer population.

2 Bisphosphonates, e.g. risedronate and alendronate, work by binding to hydroxyapatite in the bone thus inhibiting bone resorption. Effects seen in the first 12–18 months of use. Both shown to increase bone mass of the spine and the hip and to reduce fractures. There is a weekly preparation of alendronate, an advantage because it is taken on an empty stomach, with the patient erect to ensure absorption. Thus patients only miss their early morning cup of tea once a week! Side-effects include gastric irritation, abdominal pain, diarrhoea and constipation. Effective in the biologically younger population.

3 SERMS (selective oestrogen modulators), e.g. raloxifene, act as oestrogen agonists in the bone and liver but oestrogen antagonists in the breast and uterus and therefore increase bone density without increasing the risk of breast or uterine cancer.

4 Calcitonin: is an intramuscular injection, a useful adjunct in pain control of an acute fracture.

5 Analgesia essential for all osteoporotic fractures.

6 Treat causes of secondary osteoporosis.

7 Internal fixation of NOF.

Prevention of further fractures

- Treatment of osteoporosis.
- Exercise programs.
- Falls prevention strategies (see Chapter 5).
- Hip protector pads.

Osteomalacia

This is reduced calcification of the osteoid matrix due to vitamin D deficiency. The amount of bone is normal, but it is soft and weak compared with normal bone.

Incidence

Is uncertain and depends on population studied:

- Admissions to Scottish departments of geriatric medicine, 4%.
- Post-mortem study of elderly patients, 12%.
- Biopsies on fractured neck of femur patients, 25%.

Causes

1 Reduced vitamin D availability:
  (a) Deficient diet.
  (b) Reduced sun exposure: most common in Muslim and Hindu cultures which may shield women from the sun, and institutionalized elderly people.
  (c) Malabsorption, e.g. secondary to coeliac disease, diverticular disease of the small bowel and post-gastrectomy.

2 Impaired vitamin D metabolism:
  (a) Chronic renal failure.
  (b) Drugs which induce liver enzymes, e.g. phenytoin and carbamazepine.

Clinical features

- Pain in the axial skeleton (spine, shoulders, ribs, and pelvis).
- Muscle weakness.
- Waddling gait and difficulty standing from sitting secondary to osteomalacic myopathy.
- Fragility fractures.

Investigations

- X-rays may show insufficiency fractures, Looser's zones.
- Bone scintigram may show 'hungry bones', so called because the bones take up the isotope so readily that they are very bright and the kidneys may not be visible.
- Blood tests: raised alkaline phosphatase, low corrected calcium and low phosphate.
- Serum 25 hydroxyvitamin D3 will also be low.
- Bone biopsy will clinch the diagnosis where there is doubt.

Treatment

- Oral vitamin supplements, e.g. vitamin D and calcium.
- In the case of abnormal metabolism, e.g. renal disease, need to give alphcalcidol or calcitriol.
- Watch for hypercalcaemia.

Paget's disease of the bone

This is a localised abnormality of bone that arises because of increased activity of the osteoclasts and osteoblasts. The net result is an increase in bone turnover, which produces bone that is increased in size, but paradoxically weaker than normal bone. Paget's disease of the bone most frequently affects the pelvis, spine, skull and the femur, although any bone can be affected. A single bone is affected in 10% of cases. The adjacent bone may also be affected.

Incidence

Increases with age. The prevalence is 5% of over 40 year olds, rising to 10% of over 90 year olds.

Aetiology

This is still unknown, but there is likely to be a link between environmental and genetic factors. There have been studies linking it to parvovirus. A candidate gene has been found on chromosome 18q2. There is also a link with HLA DQW 1 antigen.

Clinical features

• It is usually asymptomatic and is diagnosed incidentally on X-rays.
• Pain, localised or secondary to nerve entrapment.
• Deformity, e.g. enlargement of the skull, anterior bowing of the tibia or lateral bowing of the femur.

Investigations

1 Raised serum alkaline phosphatase.
2 Raised urinary hydroxyproline suggest active disease.
3 Serum calcium is raised in patients who are immobile.
4 X-rays show the bones to be enlarged, abnormally dense and distorted.

Complications

• Fractures of abnormal bone.
• Secondary osteoarthritis of adjacent joints.
• Neurological: compression of the cranial

nerves as they exit the skull, most commonly affects the eighth nerve, but can also affect the second and the fifth; paraplegia.
• Hydrocephalus.
• High output heart failure very rare.
• The development of malignant tumours is also rare, but examples include osteosarcoma, and chondrosarcoma.

Treatment

• Aimed at treating pain and preventing deformities and fractures.
• Acute disease is treated with a bisphosphonate, usually risedronate, which reduces disease activity (mirrored by a fall in serum alkaline phosphatase and urinary hydroxyproline) and pain within days of starting treatment.
• Risedronate is usually given for 2–6 months.
• Treatment can be repeated if necessary.
• Intravenous pamidronate can be given if an oral preparation is not tolerated or if the disease is rapidly progressing.

Hyperparathyroidism

Incidence

• Two hundred and fifty cases per million population per year.
• Occurs worldwide.
• Fifty five per cent of cases will be women over 70 years of age.

Clinical features

• The majority of elderly patients will be asymptomatic and have been discovered on biochemical testing done for other reasons.
• Asymptomatic patients should simply be observed and their biochemistry monitored.
• However, 12% of cases with a raised calcium level will have had documented episodes of confusion and dehydration and will merit treatment if otherwise well.
• Check parathyroid-hormone level.
• A Sesta MIBI scan: technetium 99 is preferentially taken up by overactive parathyroid gland(s) to demonstrate the anatomy prior to surgery.
• Minimally invasive parathyroidectomy is now available.

Hypercalcaemia

There are many causes of hypercalcaemia. In practice, the following are the main groups affecting older people:

- Primary hyperparathyroidism as above.
- The hypercalcaemia of malignancy may be due to bone metastases but also non-metastatic manifestation of malignant disease.
- Myeloma, see Chapter 14.
- Drug-induced: thiazide diuretics, lithium, and vitamin D.
- Renal failure, see Chapter 13.
- Sarcoidosis, hyperthyroidism and Addison's disease are rare causes in this age group.

Emergency treatment involves rehydration with intravenous normal saline plus loop diuretics if there is fluid overload. Intravenous pamidronate is an effective treatment especially in malignancy.

Joints

To many people joint problems seem to be part of growing older — but arthritis is not universal and in old age it must be as precisely diagnosed as possible in order that appropriate treatment and management may be instigated (Table 6.1).

Osteoarthritis

- Osteoarthritis is the most common joint disorder and the incidence increases with increasing age.
- Three-quarters of people over the age of 65 years have some X-ray evidence of osteoarthritis.
- Two-thirds of people over the age of 65 years have symptoms from osteoarthritis.
- Small changes in management may produce big improvements in quality of life and symptom control.

- Joint abnormalities arise because of failure of normal repair of cartilage and periarticular bone after injury, leading to damage of the cartilage and abnormal new bone formation, such as osteophytes and secondary changes in the synovium.
- Long-standing, complicated and burnt-out rheumatoid arthritis may be difficult to differentiate from generalized osteoarthritis in old age.
- Aetiology usually unknown, i.e. primary osteoarthritis.
- May be secondary to:
  (a) Genetic predisposition.
  (b) Repetitive heavy loading of the joints.
  (c) Obesity.
  (d) Trauma leading to articular deformity.
  (e) Inflammatory disease, including gout and rheumatoid arthritis.
  (f) Aseptic necrosis.
  (g) Endocrine disease, e.g. myxoedema and acromegaly.
  (h) Neuropathic, e.g. diabetic and therefore painless.
  (i) Hereditary disease, e.g. haemophilia.
  (j) Metabolic disease, e.g. Wilson's disease, haemochromatosis, homocysteinuria.

Symptoms

- Pain: gradual in onset, intermittent, worse on movement and relieved by rest.
- Sleep may be disturbed in severe cases.
- Joints most often affected are DIPs, PIPs, base of thumb (painless but unsightly), hips, knees and cervical and lumbar spine.
- Hip pain is worse in the anterior groin and may be radiating into the buttock or thigh.
- Knee pain worse in the anterior knee and patellofemoral joint, but may be referred to the hip.
- Early morning stiffness for less than 15 min.

JOINT DISEASES: CONSULTING RATE					
All ages	0–14	15–44	45–64	65–74	75+
34	2	14	62	105	114

Table 6.1 Patient consulting rate per 1000 persons (by age in years) for patients with joint diseases.

• Functional problems include difficulty bending down to put on shoes, getting out of a chair, walking long distances which eventually may lead to immobility.

Signs
• Tenderness and bony swelling secondary to osteophytes and swelling due to effusion.
• Painful, reduced range of movement.
• In osteoarthritis of the hip, the leg may be shortened because the hip is flexed and externally rotated and there may be marked quadriceps wasting.
• Crepitus.
• Eventually the joint may become deformed, e.g. genu valgus and varus, bunion.
• Gait may be antalgic, i.e. less time is spent with weight on the affected side.

Treatment
Pharmacological
• Simple analgesia, such as paracetamol taken regularly can be enough to control pain.
• NSAIDs should be reserved for flare-ups because of multiple side effects. COX-2 inhibitors, such as rofecoxib and celecoxib, are designed to preferentially treat inflammation without causing GI symptoms, but it is still too early to evaluate their use fully.
• Capsaicin applied topically can give good pain relief.
• Intra-articular steroid injection can produce pain relief for a period of 2 weeks, sufficient to allow a patient to enjoy a special occasion, but is not indicated for long-term treatment.

Non-pharmacological
• Weight loss relieves the strain on the joints.
• Physiotherapy is aimed at improving the range of movement, strengthening muscles surrounding the joint and thus stabilising the joint.
• Using a stick in the opposite hand or a frame can reduce the load on an affected hip or knee by 50%.
• Hot and cold packs for temporary relief of pain.
• Joint replacement.

The ideal patient for joint replacement

• Refractory pain in single joint or only one severely affected joint
• Physically fit
• Well motivated
• Mentally alert and orientated
• Well nourished, but not obese
• Unlikely to place unreasonable demands on new hip, i.e. normal mobility anticipated post-operatively and not excessive activity
• Of sufficient age so that patient is unlikely to outlive the new joint. About one-quarter of replacement hips need revision after 10 years

---

Complications of joint replacement
• Infection: affects about 1% of hip replacements. Usually prophylactic antibiotics are given. The most common infection is a simple wound infection but a deeper infection may be more difficult to diagnose; a gallium scan might be helpful.
• DVT: subcutaneous low molecular weight heparin is usually given as prophylaxis.
• Loosening of prosthesis: X-ray or bone scan may demonstrate.
• Fracture of adjacent bone: visible on X-ray.
• Patient outlives prosthesis and second operation needed.
• Increased mobility reveals another pathology, e.g. angina results from the increased activity.

Rheumatoid arthritis
• *Inactive disease*—an episode in earlier life which has burnt itself out but leaving many deformities and disabilities, sometimes progressing to a mixture of old rheumatoid arthritis and more recent osteoarthritis. Treatment as for osteoarthritis (see above).
• *Active disease*—arising in old age for the first time can be difficult to differentiate from polymyalgia rheumatica.
• *Exacerbation of old disease.*

Active disease

- May have very sudden and severe onset in old age
- May be self-limiting
- Equal sex incidence (females no longer predominate)
- Fewer systemic complications
- Treatment may be more hazardous in old age

Potential problems in the treatment of rheumatoid arthritis in elderly patients.

- *Splinting* — if bulky and heavy, may significantly interfere with frail person's ability to maintain personal independence. Night splints are acceptable to some patients.
- *Rehabilitation* — the presence of severe upper-limb problems and other disorders will significantly hinder a patient's ability to co-operate fully in an intensive physiotherapy programme.
- *Drugs* — are often dangerous in old age, but important and valuable:

   (a) Quick symptom relief may be the best way to preserve mobility and independence; therefore steroids (in spite of disadvantages) may be used earlier than in younger patients.

   (b) Disease modifying anti-rheumatic drugs (DMARDS) may act too slowly to benefit older people. Also, there is increased risk of side effects because of age and pathological changes in other systems, e.g. renal impairment worsened by penicillamine and gold, visual impairment potentiated by chloroquine. The role of the anti-tumour necrosis factor agents, such as infliximab has not been assessed in the older population.

   (c) Main-line treatment in active disease is NSAIDs, but all complications of treatment are more pronounced in the elderly.

   (d) COX-2 inhibitors inhibit synovial prostaglandins without inhibiting intestinal prostaglandins thus relatively sparing the GI tract.

Crystal arthropathy

Sudden severe pain causing immobility due to acute inflammatory response. All causes are age-related and sex incidence in old age approaches equality (Table 6.2).

NB: Both gout and pseudogout may be confused with acute joint sepsis. Aspiration for pus and crystals is the best technique for differentiation.

Infective arthropathy

- Should be considered when a single joint is painful.
- Difficult to diagnose in presence of old joint deformities.
- May be confused with gout or pseudogout.
- Systemic toxic effects may be minimal in the elderly.
- Concurrent treatment may mask the problem, e.g. steroids, analgesics and antibiotics.
- Aspirate if in doubt.

Muscle pain

Polymyalgia rheumatica

Generalized muscle pain and tenderness. Probably due to an arteritis and linked with giant-cell arteritis — usually idiopathic, but may be triggered by a viral infection or may indicate the presence of an underlying malignancy.

Epidemiology

- Most common in people aged 60–70.
- Male to female ratio is 2 : 1.
- Incidence is 20/100 000 p.a.
- It is the most common reason for commencing older people on steroids.

Diagnostic criteria

1 Bilateral shoulder pain and/or neck stiffness.
2 Onset of illness of less than 2 weeks.
3 Initial ESR greater than 40.
4 Duration of morning stiffness of more than 1 h.
5 Age greater than 65 years.
6 Depression and/or weight loss.
7 Bilateral tenderness in upper arms.

Three positives are suggestive of polymyalgia rheumatica. Those features higher in the list are most strongly predictive of polymyalgia rheumatica. A successful therapeutic trial with steroids will confirm diagnosis : the response is often dramatic.

CRYSTAL ARTHROPATHY

Gout	Pseudogout
Urate crystals	Pyrophosphate crystals
Usually the great toe affected	Usually the knee is affected
May be precipitated by: Diuretics Overindulgence Fasting Excessive exercise or rest Acute illness or surgery Secondary to blood malignancies	No clear precipitation—but acute illness or surgery may be responsible
Tophi may be present	Chondrocalcinosis may be present
Uric acid level raised	Uric acid may be normal
NSAIDs and specific treatment: Colchicine Probenecid Allopurinol	Anti-inflammatory treatment only
Erosion on X-ray	Chondrocalcinosis on X-ray
Obesity, increased blood pressure and ischaemic heart disease are associated conditions	Diabetes, hyperparathyroidism, myxoedema are associated conditions
Family history common	Family history less common

Table 6.2 Clinical features, precipitating factors and treatment of crystal arthropathies.

NB: Creatinine phosphokinase, muscle biopsy and EMG are all usually normal.

Complications of untreated polymyalgia rheumatica
• Chronic disability.
• Normochromic anaemia.
• Hepatitis with raised alkaline phosphatase.
• The patient may become immobile.
• Progression to giant-cell arteritis with major vessel occlusion, leading to blindness, stroke or myocardial infarction.

Treatment
1 Steroids: 20 mg prednisolone daily for polymyalgia rheumatica, higher doses if giant cell arthritis is suspected. Rapid improvement in symptoms helps to confirm the diagnosis.
2 Dosage should be monitored according to symptoms and elevation of ESR.
3 Bone protection should be given. Use calcium and vitamin D in older, frailer people and bisphosphonates in biologically fitter people.
4 Treatment may be necessary for 2 years or more and disease may recur and require more steroids.
5 Symptoms may be relieved by NSAIDs but they will not protect the patient from vascular occlusion.

Muscle weakness

Ageing changes
Muscle bulk and effectiveness decline with increasing age. Musculature becomes atrophic and paler in colour due to a decrease in muscle fibres, an increase in fat and fibrous tissue and increased deposition of lipochrome pigment.

These changes are not exclusively due to ageing, but merely reflect the more sedentary life in old age in developed countries—muscle bulk can still be increased in the elderly by regular exercise. Neuronal impairment may be another explanation for the 'ageing changes'.

Muscle pathology in old age

Myositis
• Tender and weak muscles.
• Rarely infective in old age, but transient postviral symptoms are common.
• Often associated with underlying malignancy.
• Often associated with skin involvement—dermatomyositis.

Myopathy
• Weak muscles usually proximal and without tenderness.
• Non-metastatic complication of malignancy commonest cause.
• Endocrine—Cushing's; thyrotoxicosis; diabetes mellitus—amyotrophy.
• Drug-induced, e.g. statins, steroids and alcohol.
• Metabolic, usually due to hypokalaemia (endocrine- or drug-induced).
• Also vitamin D deficiency (part of osteomalacia).

Myasthenia
• Exaggerated fatiguability; 10% of all cases occur in old age.
• Idiopathic—corrected by edrophonium chloride (Tensilon®).
• May be associated with underlying malignancy—poor response to Tensilon®.

• May be drug-induced (penicillamine and aminoglycosides).

Investigation of muscle disease
1 Raised creatinine phosphokinase indicates muscle damage.
2 An EMG helps differentiate neurogenic and primary muscle disorders.
3 Biopsy—difficult and requires skilled and experienced interpretation; therefore best results from specialized centres.
4 Tensilon® test—in suspected myasthenia.
5 Specific tests to confirm underlying cause, e.g. thyroid-function tests.

Treatment
• Correct precipitating cause, if possible.
• Anticholinesterases in myasthenia.
• Steroids worth trying in malignant myopathy, especially polymyositis/dermatomyositis, but beware of causing steroid myopathy.

Further information

Hamerman, D. (ed.) (1988) *Clinics in Geriatric Medicine—Rheumatic Disorders.* W.B. Saunders, Philadelphia.

Misbah, S.A. (ed.) (2001) *Rheumatology and Clinical Immunology.* In: *Medical Masterclass* (Firth, J.D. ed. in chief). Blackwell Science, Oxford.

Perry, H.M. (1994) *Clinics in Geriatric Medicine—The Ageing Skeleton.* W.B. Saunders, Philadelphia.

Wright, V. (ed.) (1983) *Bone Disease in the Elderly.* Churchill Livingstone, Edinburgh.

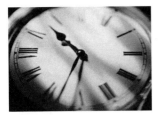

Stroke Made Simple

Importance

Anyone can have a stroke, including babies and children, but the vast majority — nine out of 10 — affect people aged over 55. Each year over 100 000 people in England and Wales have a first stroke and stroke is the third most common cause of death, after heart disease and cancer. Stroke is the largest single cause of severe disability in developed countries and is very expensive as patients need prolonged rehabilitation and, sometimes, care for life. Managing stroke in a stroke unit (multi-disciplinary, co-ordinated care) produces marked benefit — of every 16 stroke patients admitted to a general ward, there would be one extra death compared with a stroke unit.

Definition

A stroke or cerebrovascular accident (CVA) is defined as 'rapidly developing clinical signs of focal (or global) disturbance of cerebral function, with symptoms lasting 24 hours or longer or leading to death, with no apparent cause other than of vascular origin'. This includes sub-arachnoid haemorrhage (SAH) but excludes subdural haematoma (SDH) and haemorrhage into a tumour. By definition, a transient is-chaemic attack (TIA) lasts less than 24 h and so TIAs are classified separately, but the causes of TIA and stroke are very similar and TIAs are a risk factor for stroke.

Outcome of stroke

The outcome of a stroke (Table 7.1) depends on the volume and part of brain that is affected, the fitness of the patient and co-existing conditions. You will see a range of figures for outcome, depending on the population in the study, but overall the rule of thirds is useful: one third make a good recovery, one third die and one third suffer residual impairment, disability and handicap (about one half, moderate and one half severe).

Aetiology and pathology

A stroke results from interruption to the brain's blood supply due to an infarct or a haemorrhage. An infarct is an area of ischaemia (usually due to thrombosis *in situ* or an embolus from the carotids or heart but occasionally due to low blood pressure from any cause or damage to the blood vessel wall). A primary haemorrhage may be due to an arterial abnormality, such as an aneurysm, but both infarcts and bleeds usually occur in vessels damaged by hypertension and atheroma. Sometimes there is secondary bleeding into an area of brain damaged by an infarct. The proportions of the types of stroke vary in different countries. In the UK atherothrombotic strokes comprise 80%, in Japan, haemorrhagic strokes are much commoner. The biggest risk factor for stroke is increasing age but it is more useful to consider risk factors that can be treated.

Risk factors for stroke are similar to those for other vascular disease such as ischaemic heart disease (IHD) and peripheral vascular disease (Table 7.2). However, there are differences in relative risk that are not understood, e.g. smoking is a bigger risk for IHD and hypertension is a bigger risk for stroke. In future, more may be understood about the role of inflammation as high CRP (though still within the 'normal range') is emerging as a risk factor for vascular disease. In general, primary and secondary risk factors are similar. Risk factors tend to multiply. As there

OUTCOME OF STROKE

1-month mortality	25–50%
1-year mortality of survivors	40%
Full or almost full recovery	25–50%
Return to work if previously working	30–35%
Unable to walk outdoors	40%
Unable to walk unaided	20–25%
Long-term high-dependency care	12–20%

Table 7.1.

PRIMARY AND SECONDARY RISK FACTORS

Risk factor	Management	Goal
BP high	Promote healthy lifestyle; diet (see below), moderate alcohol intake; and exercise. Treat BP if still high with drugs individualized to other patient characteristics (e.g. age, race, need for drugs with specific benefits), but ACE inhibitors may have a particular role	<140/90 mm/Hg; <130/85 mm/Hg if renal insufficiency or heart failure is present; or <130/80 mm/Hg if diabetic
Heart disease	As appropriate for the condition, also aiming to reduce platelet stickiness, minimize development of LVH and maintain in sinus rhythm	Reduce chances of embolization
Atrial fibrillation	Verify AF on ECG. Convert to sinus rhythm if possible. For patients in chronic or intermittent AF, use warfarin aiming for INR 2.0–3.0 (target 2.5). Aspirin is used if there are contraindications to oral anticoagulation. Low-risk patients <65 years may be treated with aspirin	Sinus rhythm: anti-platelet treatment or anticoagulation if AF persists
Plaque formation (platelets adhere)	Aspirin except in aspirin intolerance and brain haemorrhage, caution with asthma and history of GI haemorrhage. Consider 75–300 mg aspirin per day for persons at higher vascular risk	Low-dose aspirin in persons at higher vascular risk; consider clopidogrel if intolerant or adding modified-release dipyridamole
Carotid stenosis	Anti-platelet therapy, document degree of stenosis and offer endarterectomy if CT confirms stroke in opposite hemisphere, function worth preserving and stenosis >70% or >50% if over 75 years	Ensure eligible patients with anterior circulation strokes are screened: the fit elderly have most to gain

Table 7.2 Primary and secondary risk factors for stroke.

PRIMARY AND SECONDARY RISK FACTORS (*Cont.*)

Risk factor	Management	Goal
Smoking	Check smoking status, advise quitting and refer for support, e.g. clinic/pharmacological help (nicotine or buproprion)	Quit and avoid passive smoking
Unhealthy diet	Advocate low fat, low salt, high fruit and vegetable diet with weight loss if needed. Discourage excess consumption of any food however 'healthy' to avoid health scares, e.g. heavy metals in oily fish	Varied healthy diet
Obesity	Calorie restriction and increased caloric expenditure	Achieve and maintain desirable weight (BMI 18–25 kg/m²). Higher BMI is less of a risk if central obesity is not present
Excess alcohol	Low/moderate alcohol intake protects from atherothrombotic stroke (amount probably depends on individual as increase in BP and obesity may be adverse) but high or binge intake is a risk for haemorrhage	Avoid binge or excessive drinking
Adverse lipid profile	If LDL-C is above goal range, modify diet, weight and exercise. If it remains high, check liver function, thyroid function and urinalysis and consider a statin. After LDL-C goal has been reached, consider triglyceride level: persevere with diet or fibrate	LDL-C reduction is most important and the more other co-existing risk factors, the more stringent the goal
Diabetes and impaired glucose tolerance	After diet and exercise, second-step therapy is usually oral hypoglycemic drugs: sulphonylureas and/or metformin with ancillary use of acarbose and thiazolidinediones. Then consider insulin	Normal fasting plasma glucose (<7 mmol/L) and near normal HbA1c (<7%)
Lack of exercise	Medical check before initiating vigorous exercise programme: start slowly if older or unfit. Moderate-intensity activities (40–60% of maximum capacity) are equivalent to a brisk walk. Additional benefit from vigorous (>60% of maximum capacity) exercise for 20–40 min on 3–5 days/week	At least 30 min of moderate-intensity physical activity on most days of the week
Previous TIA	Treat all risk factors	

Table 7.2 *Continued.*

is more chance of another vascular event once one has occurred, the risk:benefit ratio for treatments changes. (This is why healthy 40 year olds are advised not to take aspirin as their chance of a bleed outweighs likely benefits).

Presentation

Typically, the onset is abrupt. Occasionally a hemiparesis develops over a period of 12 or more hours but, if it progresses over days or a week or two, a space-occupying lesion (SOL), such as a tumour or subdural, should be suspected. Other conditions, which may mimic stroke, are hypoglycaemia and Todd's (post-epileptic) paresis.

A stroke may present as coma of unknown cause, in which case any neurological examination requiring co-operation is impossible. The cheek on the paralysed side may flap in and out with respiration and the limbs on that side are likely to have completely lost all tone. The reflexes may be unhelpful at this stage. One finding which, if present, pretty well wraps up the diagnosis is conjugate deviation of gaze towards the side of the lesion, due to the unopposed effect of the contralateral frontal eye field. Loss of consciousness points towards a severe stroke, but by no means inevitably towards cerebral haemorrhage as the pathology.

The conscious or slightly drowsy patient, on the other hand, usually presents little diagnostic difficulty. The peak time of onset for stroke is in the early hours of the morning and, if capable of speech, the patient will describe waking up and trying to get out of bed, only to find him or herself unable to walk. An eyewitness may relate that in the middle of a meal the patient dropped his or her cup and developed facial asymmetry and difficulty with speech and then became unable to stand or perhaps even sit properly. Examination will then usually reveal characteristic deficits: in the early stages, the paralysed limbs are more often flaccid than spastic and in some cases they stay that way.

Clinical types of stroke

Transient ischaemic attacks

These are isolated or recurrent focal neurological symptoms attributed to platelet emboli from an atheromatous plaque or ulcer in the aorta, the common carotid artery or, most often, the carotid bifurcation. Monocular loss of vision (amaurosis fugax) hemi- or monoparesis, dysphasia and unilateral sensory disturbance are examples within the internal carotid territory. The problem must resolve within 24 h to be called a TIA, but most last less than a couple of hours. The distinction between a TIA and a very

small infarct is somewhat academic. Twelve per cent of patients with TIA will have a stroke within 12 months, with the greatest risk in the 1st month, and so rapid referral for Doppler duplex imaging or magnetic resonance angiography is mandatory for subjects suitable for endarterectomy.

TIAs also occur within the territory of the vertebrobasilar circulation, although vertebrobasilar ischaemia or insufficiency has been something of a diagnostic dustbin. The main features are true vertigo (a sensation of rotary movement of either patient or surroundings), true drop attacks (sudden falls due to total loss of tone without disturbance of consciousness and with rapid and complete recovery) and diplopia, although cortical blindness, tetraparesis, ataxia and dysphagia may also occur. Vertebrobasilar insufficiency does not require intervention other than aspirin.

The established stroke

Detailed descriptions of the enormous variety of syndromes explicable in terms of the precise anatomy of the damage sustained are beyond the scope of this book. The identification of the major deficits is more important and the classification devised by Bamford in 1991 (Table 7.3) is simple and provides useful prognostic information.

Clinical problems following stroke

- *Dysphagia*. Difficulty with swallowing is common initially (see Management of the established stroke, pp. 62–65).
- *Dysphasia*. Disorder of language affecting some right-handed patients with left-hemisphere lesions:

   (a) Anterior dysphasia — non-fluent, impaired naming.

   (b) Posterior dysphasia — often fluent, jargon type, receptive dysphasia.

Fluent dysphasia is often confused with 'acute confusion'! In left-handers, two-thirds have left-sided speech dominance; those who have right-sided dominance may/may not develop dysphasia, irrespective of side of lesion.
- *Dysarthria*. Disorder of articulation in which

BRAIN INFARCTION

	Clinical	Anatomy/pathology	Outcome
TACI 15%	Higher cerebral dysfunction (e.g. dysphasia, dyscalculia, visuospatial disorder) *and* hemianopia *and* ipsilateral motor *and/or* sensory deficit involving 2 out of 3 of face, arm or leg	MCA occluded by embolus/spreading thrombus from ICA	Very poor chance of good function and high mortality
PACI 35%	2/3 TACI components *or* higher cerebral dysfunction alone *or* restricted motor/sensory deficit (e.g. one limb or face, hand, not whole arm)	Branch of MCA or ACA	Fair outcome but very high chance of early recurrence
LacI 25%	Pure motor, pure sensory or sensorimotor or 'ataxic hemiparesis'	Lipohyalinosis of deep perforating artery	Often good recovery
POCI 25%	Cranial nerve palsy with contralateral motor/sensory deficit *or* bilateral motor/sensory deficits *or* dysconjugate eye movements *or* cerebellar deficit/hemianopia	Brain stem, cerebellum or occipital lobes	High chance of good function but also of recurrence in 1st year

ACA, anterior cerebral artery; ICA, internal carotid artery; LacI, lacunar infarct; MCA, middle cerebral artery; PACI, partial anterior circulatory infarct; POCI, posterior circulatory infarct; TACI, total anterior circulatory infarct.

Table 7.3 Brain infarction. (*Source*: Bamford 1991.)

the content of the speech is unaffected. This can be due to unilateral VII palsy but otherwise suggests bilateral disease (or pathology in the cerebellum or basal ganglia).
• *Dyspraxia*. Inability to perform purposeful movement despite adequate comprehension and motor function. Varieties such as dressing apraxia.
• *Sensory neglect*. Visual—exclude hemianopia first. Test by line bisection, line cancellation (Albert's test). Tactile, if gross, includes loss of body image and denial of problem.
• *Visuospatial perception*. Non-dominant hemisphere lesion—draw house, face, clock face.
• *Weakness of limbs*. Usually develop increased

tone, marked 'clasp-knife' spasticity and flaccidity are both adverse.
• *Sensory loss*. Any modality, gross-position sense loss is highly adverse.
• *Hemianopia*. Major handicap unless patient aware and able to compensate by turning head.
• *Depression*. Especially in dominant-hemisphere lesion. Treat with antidepressants.
• *Thalamic pain*. Try antidepressant or anticonvulsant.
• *Shoulder pain*. Subluxation especially likely following traction on the weak arm.

Multi-infarct disease

This condition is also known as 'lacunar state' and is seen in arteriopaths and those with atrial fibrillation (AF). The features are shown below.

Features of multi-infarct disease

- History of hypertension, etc.
- Stepwise progression
- Neurological signs depending on location
- Dementia when lacunae total 50–100 ml
- Abnormal gait *marche à petits pas*, broad-based backward-leaning
- Pseudobulbar palsy:
  - (a) Dysarthria
  - (b) Dysphagia
  - (c) Emotional lability

CT OF DIFFERENT STROKES

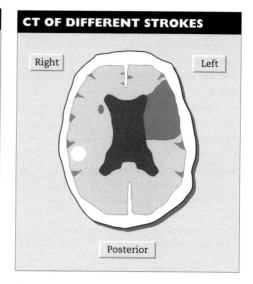

Fig. 7.1 Diagram of head CT showing appearances of a parietal haematoma and a deep lacunar infarct on the right and a total anterior circulatory infarct on the left.

Cerebellar haematoma

Requires special mention because of:

1 The axiom: 'stroke somewhere–stroke nowhere = stroke in the cerebellum' (or, it should be added, thalamus, especially if there is a severe memory deficit).

2 The fact that surgical evacuation is often beneficial, and biologically fit patients should be discussed with the neurosurgeons.

Spinal-cord infarction

This may cause sudden paraplegia or quadriplegia and is often caused by a compressing lesion. Spinal-cord ischaemia can cause 'neurogenic claudication' and mimic peripheral vascular disease.

Investigation of stroke

Typical tests may include: FBC, CRP, glucose, renal liver and bone function, cardiac enzymes if concomitant MI is possible (troponin appears more cardio-specific than CK-MB), cholesterol and thyroid function, ECG, CXR, cardiac echocardiogram and 24-h tape if cardiogenic embolus is suspected, and carotid Doppler studies.

Most stroke patients merit head CT, with the possible exception of those patients who appear so likely to die that any intervention at all seems unjustified. The area of low attenuation characteristic of an infarct often does not become apparent for up to 24 h or more. Haemorrhage is immediately apparent as a white area (Fig. 7.1).

Indications for CT for stroke patients

1 Suspicion of SOL:
  (a) Atypical presentation
  (b) Head injury
  (c) Known malignancy
2 Suspicion of SAH
3 Suspicion of meningitis
4 Need to distinguish infarct from haemorrhage (most common indication as almost always determines treatment)
5 Possible cerebellar haematoma

Management of the established stroke

Where?

Patients with minor stroke can be managed at home, providing there is sufficient family support and adequate community rehabilitation. Most, however, are admitted to hospital, mainly for nursing support. Whatever the setting, proper diagnosis (usually brain CT) and full identification of risk factors and initiation of measures for secondary prevention are essential. Even in the early phase, management of a stroke patient is multi-disciplinary.

If the patient is admitted to hospital, the outcome is much better if the patient is managed on a **stroke unit**. It is unclear which component of stroke unit care leads to the improved outcome but stroke units have been the most important advance in stroke in the last decade. Thereafter, rehabilitation can take place in the patient's own home, in a community hospital or in a day hospital, depending on circumstances.

The unconscious patient

Will need full nursing care with particular attention to airway, pressure areas, hydration and bladder drainage.

The immobile patient

Thromboembolic device stockings (TEDS) may be beneficial. Although subcutaneous heparin reduces deaths from PE, haemorrhagic deaths are increased so heparin is usually not used. Correct positioning and chest physiotherapy are needed.

Dispersing the thrombus

Unless there is a strong clinical suspicion of a bleed, give aspirin (300 mg) acutely. Trials of thrombolysis have shown benefit in very selected patients when given soon after stroke onset. More patients suffer intracranial haemorrhage but overall fewer have severe disability at 3 months. Intravenous recombinant tissue-type plasminogen (rt-PA) activator is approved by the US Food and Drug Administration for treating acute ischaemic stroke within 3 h of onset of symptoms. Post-marketing data suggest that the risk of intracranial haemorrhage may be unacceptably high when rt-PA is given to patients who would not have been eligible for enrollment in the clinical trials. Practical problems include getting patients to hospital, CT scanned within the timeframe and interpretation of the early scans.

Vasodilatation and cerebral oedema

No convincing advantage has emerged from various trials of vasodilators, partly because the vessels in the infarcted zone are already maximally dilated. The same applies to various agents designed to relieve cerebral oedema. Trials of haemodilution have also been unsuccessful.

Neuroprotection

In a stroke there is a central zone of irreversibly damaged cells surrounded by a penumbra of ischaemic but potentially salvageable cells. These face a number of threats including oedema, the release of glutamate, aspartate and lactate and an influx of calcium ions. The penumbral tissue increases its oxygen extraction (normally about 40%) from the available blood for a day or two after the event, indicating the time-scale available for intervention. Trials of N-methyl-D-aspartate (NMDA) receptor blockers, which prevent the released glutamate from causing a toxic influx of calcium ions into the neurons, have been disappointing. This may be an example of poor extrapolation from animal work to the clinical situation: glutamate does kill neurons immediately after brain injury, but preserves endangered neurons in the long term. The only way to provide neuroprotection with NMDA antagonists would be to administer them before the insult and for a very short period (minutes) after the injury, which is impossible in a stroke.

General care

Complications, such as DVT, PE, pressure sores and chest infection, are treated in the usual way.

Hydration and nutrition

There are four situations in which taking fluid and nutrition becomes a problem:
1 The unconscious or drowsy patient (transient).
2 Pseudobulbar palsy due to bilateral stroke (often prolonged).
3 Brain-stem stroke with bulbar involvement (sometimes prolonged).
4 The common hemisphere infarct (usually transient) (about 40%).

It is usual to put the patient on a nil-by-mouth regime until the patient's swallow has been assessed by the speech and language therapist. Inadequate airway protection does not equate with an absent gag reflex, nor is the reverse true.

The ability to swallow fluids is assessed by sitting the patient up and observing his or her ability to swallow a teaspoon (5 ml), a tablespoon (15 ml) and then 50–100 ml of water. Sensitivity of this observation is improved by monitoring the oxygen saturation during the procedure. If the patient is unable to swallow, pooling occurs in the mouth. Choking and obvious aspiration with coughing may ensue but some patients aspirate 'silently', which is where monitoring the oxygen saturation is helpful. Fluid and electrolytes are given intravenously. One advantage of this route is that eventually the line 'tissues', which provides an opportunity to decide whether or not to resite it. In other words, in a patient who is clearly doing very badly, it may be felt that it is best to allow nature to take its course. Fluid (usually about a litre a day) may also be given subcutaneously.

It is not permissible to procrastinate indefinitely and sooner or later the decision must be taken whether to feed as well as to hydrate the persistently dysphagic patient. The usual practice is to offer nutrition via a fine-bore nasogastric (NG) tube at 72 h after the stroke. Again it is rare for an NG tube to remain in place for more than a few days as they are easily dislodged. If the swallow still fails to recover, a percutaneous endoscopic gastrostomy (PEG) tube may be considered usually at around 10–14 days but this procedure should not be undertaken lightly as such tubes usually remain in place and raise medico-legal problems if withdrawal is considered. Remember, the purpose of feeding tubes is to nourish and hydrate, not to protect the airway; they do not prevent aspiration of contaminated oral secretions or regurgitated gastric contents. This needs to be explained to many nurses as well as the family. Decisions about hydration and feeding are difficult ethically, particularly after a stroke. Always seek senior advice.

Information for the family or patient

Depending on the severity of the stroke the patient and or the family need appropriate information. Leaflets from a patient-based society such as the Stroke Association are very helpful.

If the patient is not doing well, the team should make a decision about whether to attempt cardio-pulmonary resuscitation in the event of cardio-respiratory arrest. This is a clinical decision based on the patient's condition. It may be possible to discuss this with the patient or find out from the family what they feel the patient would have wanted. In the context of a major stroke, CPR is most unlikely to be successful. If recovery is very poor, end-of-life decisions, such as the futility of repeated antibiotic treatment should be discussed.

Rehabilitation

The 1st week of stabilization of the stroke is followed by 2–3 weeks of rapid recovery and then a further 6 months of slow but continuing improvement. Although the impairment may only achieve a further 10% of recovery during this phase, the resultant disabilities can often take longer and therefore show greater late improvement. The multi-disciplinary aspects of rehabilitation are discussed in Chapter 2.

The sequence of sitting, transferring, standing and walking may therefore take a couple of months if the hemiparesis is initially quite severe. In general, proximal movements recover more than distal and lower limbs more than upper.

Indicators of poor outcome

- Severity of stroke, e.g. total anterior circulatory infarct (TACI)
- Significant cognitive impairment
- Admitted comatose
- Persistent incontinence
- Paralysis of conjugate gaze
- Neglect, persistent visuospatial perceptual disorder
- Homonomous hemianopia
- Depression and other reasons for poor motivation
- Significant associated pathology
- No grip at 3 weeks—useful hand function unlikely

Driving after a stroke

Strokes and TIAs should be notified to the Driver and Vehicle Licensing Agency and his or her insurance company by the patient. Driving may be resumed after 3 months or so, depending on the residual deficit.

Further information

Bamford, J., Sandercock, P., Dennis, M., Burn, J. & Warlow, C. (1991) Classification and natural history of clinically identifiable subtypes of cerebral infarction. *Lancet* **22** (337):1521–6.

Caplan, L.R. (2002) Treatment of patients with stroke. *Archives of Neurology* **59**(5), 703–7. (Full text available on the internet).

Cochrane library website for regularly updated stroke reviews from the Cochrane library (search the Abstracts): http://www.update-software.com/cochrane/

Ikonomidou, C. & Turski, L. (2002) Why did NMDA receptor antagonists fail clinical trials for stroke and traumatic brain injury? *The Lancet Neurology* **1**(6), 383.

Massachusetts medical students website written with the American Stroke Association: http://www.umassmed.edu/strokestop

Straus, S.E., Majumdar, S.R. & McAlister, F.A. (2002) New evidence for stroke prevention: scientific review. *Journal of the American Medical Association* **288**(11), 1388–95.

Stroke association website:
http://www.stroke.org.uk/

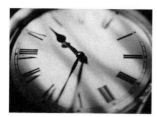

Other Diseases of the Nervous System

Age changes and clinical examination

A full examination of the CNS can be an ordeal for both a frail elderly patient and his or her doctor. Patience and understanding are required by both and compromise will often be needed.

Remember that much can be gained by simply observing the patient. The patient's memory and speech during history taking and their ability to walk to and get on to the examination couch may give you clues to underlying pathology.

Ageing changes and co-morbidities, e.g. arthritis may confuse the clinical picture. Gait changes with age, becoming slower and less regular in pattern, with feet closer together, less firm heel strike and more time with both feet on the ground. The older the patient, the more difficult the problems—almost one-third of 'normal over 80 year olds' walk with a shuffling gait and almost half have a flexed posture but most do not have Parkinson's disease (PD).

Muscle wasting is common, usually in the proximal muscles, due to disuse; this is especially a problem in very elderly women, who may find it very difficult to rise from a chair without assistance. For this reason, chairs in outpatient clinics should have arms. Wasting of the small muscles of the hand does not automatically have the sinister connotations of the same finding in young subjects.

Reflexes may be difficult to elicit because of other pathologies, e.g. osteoarthritis and ankle jerks in particular are difficult to elicit in almost one-third of elderly people. Abdominal reflexes are almost universally absent.

Pupils are often small and react sluggishly and, for these reasons, plus cataracts, examination of the fundi is often difficult or impossible (even after mydriasis).

Fine changes in sensation may be difficult to determine—moving from abnormal to normal is generally easier for patients to detect. Vibration sense is often lost or not understood, so position sense is usually a better test to employ (but fixed joints may make even this difficult).

Do be gentle with your elderly patients if you want their co-operation. If necessary, break the CNS examination down into stages and don't expect perfection from yourself or your patient.

Symptomatic classification of neurological disease in the elderly

1 *Headache*:
  (a) raised intracranial pressure but fewer than 10% of patients with brain tumour present with headache alone;
  (b) pain radiating from cervical spondylosis;
  (c) giant-cell arteritis—superficial, with tender arteries, tenderness over proximal muscles, high ESR/CRP;
  (d) psychological—but the prevalence of 'tension' headaches declines with age, consider depression;
  (e) Paget's disease of the skull is occasionally painful when active—often obvious;

(f) migraine but new onset migraine is unusual over 50 years.

2 *Pain in face:*
(a) trigeminal neuralgia—mean age of onset around 50 years, rarely starts in old age;
(b) dental problems;
(c) sinusitis;
(d) giant-cell arteritis (pain on chewing);
(e) post-herpetic neuralgia (look for post-inflammatory pigmentary change in a trigeminal dermatome).

3 *Hemiparesis:*
(a) vascular disease;
(b) space-occupying lesion;
(c) unilateral PD.

4 *Paraparesis:*
(a) cord compression—either vascular or space-occupying lesion;
(b) CSF infection ;
(c) Guillain–Barré syndrome;
(d) pressure from disc, bone or collection of pus.

5 *Unsteadiness:*
(a) neuropathy proximal myopathy;
(b) cerebellar disease;
(c) drug-induced;
(d) cerebrovascular disease;
(e) middle-ear disease;
(f) myxoedema.

6 *Rigidity/immobility:*
(a) PD;
(b) drugs—especially phenothiazines;
(c) disuse;
(d) joint/bone problems;
(e) spasticity of multi-infarct dementia.

7 *Asymmetrical weakness:*
(a) nerve entrapment;
(b) motor-neuron disease;
(c) diabetes—mononeuritis.

8 *Clouding of consciousness:*
(a) meningitis or encephalitis and sepsis at any site;
(b) raised intracranial pressure;
(c) drugs (sedatives, hypnotics);
(d) biochemical disturbances.

9 *Coma:*
(a) stroke (large lesions in the cerebral hemispheres, small lesions in the brain-stem);
(b) space-occupying lesion;
(c) fit;
(d) drugs (sedatives, hypnotics, alcohol);
(e) poisoning (accidental—remember carbon monoxide—self-harm, iatrogenic, rarely, deliberate);
(f) biochemical disturbance (hypoglycaemia is the one not to miss—check the glucose).

10 *Involuntary movement:*
(a) PD;
(b) drugs (anti-Parkinsonian treatment, neuroleptics);
(c) benign essential tremor;
(d) vascular disease (choreiform movements and hemiballismus are usually due to stroke in old age);
(e) epilepsy;
(f) cerebellar disease.

Aetiological classification

Vascular disease
See Chapter 7 for stroke and multi-infarct disease.

Trauma
Fractured skull
Fractures are important if depressed as pieces of bone may damage underlying cortex. Diplopia may indicate a fractured orbit. Fractures through a sinus or the ear may allow entry of organisms and lead to meningitis so prophylactic antibiotics are given. Fracture through the temporal bone can result in a result in an extradural haemorrhage. However, a routine X-ray of the skull after an uncomplicated fall is not justified. If an X-ray is done, fractures are hard to spot but always look for a horizontal line indicating an air/fluid (blood) level.

Subdural haematoma
This is commoner in old age because of increased frequency of falls and it is said that cerebral atrophy allows continued oozing of blood in to the subdural space. A subdural may be asymptomatic, cause mild unilateral weakness, intel-

lectual impairment, fits or loss of consciousness. A fluctuating course or disproportionate drowsiness in a patient with a hemiparesis may alert the clinician to this diagnosis. Increased use of anticoagulants in old age (e.g. for AF) exposes many patients to the risk of subdural bleeding, especially if prone to fall or drink to excess, or INR control is poor due to frequent changes in drug regime or poor compliance.

Diagnosis confirmed by head CT. The hardest decision is often whether to operate and although the appearance of the blood alters with time, it can be hard to be precise about when the subdural developed. It is difficult to predict whether drainage will improve the clinical state, particularly in dementia. Find out as much detail about the patient's prior functional performance as possible from carers or relatives and, if in doubt, ask the neurosurgeons.

Cord compression
Cord compression may be secondary to a prolapsed disc, pressure from tumour, osteophytes (especially cervical spondylosis) or collapsed vertebra (usually secondary to other pathology, from osteoporosis to malignant disease) or an epidural abscess. A fall may be the precipitating event in a patient who had asymptomatic pathology. Straight X-rays are sometimes difficult to interpret, especially in the cervical spine, where degenerative changes are very common.

A sensory level, if present, will help identify the region for further investigation; it is usually several segments below the level of cord compression. Remember that lesions in the lumbar region or lower will present with lower-motor-neuron (LMN) signs as the cord ends at L1/2 and those above with upper-motor-neuron (UMN) signs or a mixed picture, e.g. cervical spondylosis causing compression leads to LMN symptoms and signs in the arms but UMN changes in legs. Check for loss of sphincter control.

Sudden onset of cord compression is an emergency and rapid investigation is essential if active intervention (surgery or radiotherapy) is to avoid permanent damage. MRI is better than CT but the latter may be preferable if it is available faster.

Lumbar canal stenosis
This is usually due to a congenitally narrow canal but presents in middle or old age as osteophytes or a disc encroach on the cauda equina; remember the cord terminates at L2 in adults. It may produce weakness of the legs or present with a pain like intermittent claudication (better on stairs as the spine is flexed).

Normal pressure hydrocephalus
Normal pressure hydrocephalus is a condition exclusive to later life. Its cause is unknown but simplistically it is assumed that when the condition is developing some abnormality in CSF flow must at least sporadically increase the pressure. Its presentation is insidious, with a triad of intellectual failure, unsteadiness (with broad-based gait or gait apraxia) and early urinary incontinence. Diagnosis is made by CT, which will show enlarged ventricles without widened sulci. However, variation in the relative amounts of ventricular enlargement to cerebral atrophy in normal ageing and dementia make this a difficult diagnosis. By the time of diagnosis, the CSF pressure is 'normal'. It is said that treatment by shunting may be successful and some suggest that response to a lumbar puncture predicts response from the shunt. However, the procedure is rare and as there are no trials at all, Cochrane recently concluded that there was no evidence to support shunting.

Hydrocephalus may also be secondary to previous cerebral damage from episodes of bleeding (especially subarachnoid haemorrhage) or meningitis. A strategically placed space-occupying lesion in the mid-brain may also lead to hydrocephalus.

Degenerative or idiopathic disease
Parkinson's disease
An idiopathic degenerative condition with progressive death of the dopaminergic neurons of the substantia nigra (SN) in the basal ganglia. Symptoms appear when around 80% of the dopamine has been lost and are due to a lack of

dopamine and a relative excess of acetylcholine. PD is thought to occur in the genetically susceptible exposed to an environmental trigger but the nature of both components remains unknown. Rare young-onset PD has a clearer genetic component and some of the gene defects are characterized. At histological examination (post-mortem), the finding of Lewy bodies (intracytoplasmic inclusion bodies containing alpha synuclein) restricted to the SN is pathognomonic. Many cases diagnosed in life (perhaps 20%) are not confirmed as PD on post-mortem examination. The incidence increases with age (250/10^5 aged 60–69 to 2000/10^5 aged over 80).

Diagnosis
PD is always a difficult diagnosis in the early stages, especially in the very old who may 'normally' have some features of extrapyramidal rigidity. The triad of classical symptoms and signs are poverty of movement (akinesia, bradykinesia), regular tremor at rest (5/s 'pill rolling') and rigidity of extrapyramidal type ('lead pipe') or cogwheel rigidity in presence of tremor.

The tremor may be obvious and is usually a rest tremor and may be unilateral. It disappears in sleep. The bradykinesia may be apparent as paucity of facial expression (Parkinsonian facies), and difficulty with fine movements, typically doing up buttons. The handwriting may get smaller during the course of a sentence (micrographia). Speech is soft (dysphonic), monotonous and becomes dysarthric. The stiffness may be misinterpreted as arthritis and although PD does not affect the sensory sytem, the joint stiffness, particularly in bed at night may be painful. The gait is characteristic with a flexed posture, tendency to shuffle, loss of arm swing, and impaired postural reflexes which make the patient likely to fall. Stopping, starting and turning are the aspects of walking which pose most difficulty and if a walking frame is needed, a wheeled type is usually recommended. As the disease progresses, constipation, bladder instability and drooling may be troublesome.

A therapeutic trial may be helpful in confirming the diagnosis; this usually consists of oral levodopa and measuring the time to walk a set distance (10 m) or to carry out a tap test—the number of pronations and supinations the patient can achieve in a minute tapping on a desk or inspection of handwriting (micrographia should be seen to improve).

Management
All patients with PD benefit from a multi-disciplinary package of care of which drug treatment is only one component. As the disease progresses the relative emphasis of the components will change. Learn the list below—suitably modified it will provide an outline of how to manage most chronic conditions at any age, from multiple sclerosis to COPD!

Management options include:
1 *Education and support*—all patients or carers should be encouraged to join the Parkinson's Disease Society (see website: www.parkinsons.org.uk).
2 *Continuity of care*—chronic progressive diseases are best managed in settings that allow continuity of care to enable the patient and clinician to develop a working relationship and to assess the benefits and side-effects of treatment. In many areas there is a PD clinic run by a geriatrician, neurologist or both, often with a *nurse specialist*. The nurse can often visit the patient at home and provide telephone advice between appointments.
3 *Therapy*—assessment and treatment:
  (a) Physiotherapy: work on posture, gait, falls prevention.
  (b) Occupational therapy: maintaining skills, home modification, etc.
  (c) Speech and language therapy: speech production, facial expression, swallowing.
4 *Dietitian*—advice on maintaining nutrition and protein spacing.
5 *Assessment of benefits.*
6 *Legal advice*—patients should be informed about Enduring Power of Attorney, driving regulations and may wish to consider living wills, etc.
7 Maintenance of general *health and fitness.*
8 *Treat other problems*—cataracts or ingrowing toenails (refer for podiatry) do not help Parkinsonian gait.

9 Maintenance of *morale and mood* (consider complementary medicine, antidepressants).

Drugs

In the future, it is hoped to find 'neuroprotective' drugs that prevent the process that leads to cell death. Increasing evidence suggests that neurons die in PD by a process called apoptosis, which may be triggered by mitochondrial impairment and oxidative stress. Claims have been made that some of the current drugs, e.g. selegiline, may be neuroprotective but these claims are controversial. Other drugs are being tested; two novel synthetic inhibitors of the tumor suppressor protein p53, pifithrin- (PFT-) and Z-1–117, are highly effective in protecting mid-brain dopaminergic neurons and improving behavioral outcome in a mouse model of PD. There is also some evidence for benefit from co-enzyme Q10, a supplement available in health shops, but larger trials are needed.

Current drug treatment aims to restore transmitter balance in the basal ganglia:

Whilst the types of drugs available are logical (Fig. 8.1), the order in which they are prescribed varies not only with the patient but also the prescriber, i.e. the weight of evidence does not clearly support one course of action. Assuming the diagnosis is correct, levodopa preparations usually provide excellent benefits initially, but over a few years, the 'long-term levodopa syndrome' emerges. Problems may be predictable at first, for example soon after a dose there may be involuntary movements (peak dose dyskinesia) and as the next dose becomes due, the effect of the previous dose may wear off so that the patient becomes rigid, immobile and frozen or 'off'. These effects can be ameliorated by careful juggling of doses and timing but eventually the fluctuations can become severe, sometimes random and the patient may alternate between being 'on' for short periods only with 'offs' and disabling dyskinesias. There is some evidence that the duration or dose × years of levodopa treatment affects the development of this syndrome, perhaps because of pulsatile stimulation

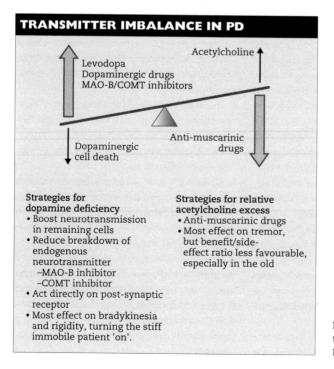

TRANSMITTER IMBALANCE IN PD

Levodopa
Dopaminergic drugs
MAO-B/COMT inhibitors

Acetylcholine

Dopaminergic cell death

Anti-muscarinic drugs

Strategies for dopamine deficiency
• Boost neurotransmission in remaining cells
• Reduce breakdown of endogenous neurotransmitter
  –MAO-B inhibitor
  –COMT inhibitor
• Act directly on post-synaptic receptor
• Most effect on bradykinesia and rigidity, turning the stiff immobile patient 'on'.

Strategies for relative acetylcholine excess
• Anti-muscarinic drugs
• Most effect on tremor, but benefit/side-effect ratio less favourable, especially in the old

Fig. 8.1 Strategies for treating the transmitter imbalance in Parkinson's disease.

of the receptors. In younger patients the long-acting agonists are increasingly used as the first-line drugs. There is less information in older people but, particularly if the PD is already impacting on function when the diagnosis is made, many doctors still tend to give levodopa. The dose of levodopa is more often limited by neuropsychiatric problems (confusion, hallucinations) than dyskinesia, which is the case in the middle aged.

Associated problems relating to bladder, bowels, digestion, sleep and mood often complicate PD. It is debatable as to whether these are all part of the complete picture or simply common accompaniments to chronic disease and disability. To the patients it doesn't matter and all such problems need to be helped by drug treatment or lifestyle changes. Although in theory SSRIs could worsen PD, they are usually used but with caution if the patient is on selegiline.

The most significant complication of PD is the associated dementia, which is common in elderly patients. It may seriously limit the patient's ability to continue with levodopa treatment. Neurologists once told Parkinson's patients that they would die **with** PD, not **from** it. However, the terminal stages of PD in old age are distressing, the patient being robbed of mobility, cognitive function, swallowing and sphincter control. Enormous amounts of support to both carers and patients are required at this distressing stage. Support at earlier times is also needed and often most frequently supplied by contact with the Parkinson's Disease Society.

Experimental forms of treatment available in a few specialist centres are not usually recommended for/available to frail older patients. These include neurosurgery—pallidotomy (for contralateral dyskinesias) has seen a resurgence and deep-brain stimulation may help severe tremor. Transplantation of fetal adrenal tissue has not fulfilled its expectations but may eventually become a reality with cultured cells, once fundamental issues such as how to 'turn off' the dopamine production from transplanted cells have been solved. A promising area is infusion of glial-derived neurotrophic factor, which is undergoing early clinical trials.

Parkinsonism

There are a number of causes for a Parkinsonian syndrome:

1 *Drugs*—the most frequent being the neuroleptics, the saddest of which is prochloperazine; Parkinsonism is a devastating sequel to a usually ineffectual prescription for 'dizziness'.
2 *Virus*—post-encephalitic
3 *Toxins*—PD induced by contaminated illegal drugs—MPTP (1-methyl-4-phenyl-1,2,3,4-tetrahydropyridine) and, more worryingly, case reports associated with Ecstasy.
4 *Trauma*—as in ex-boxers.
5 *Vascular disease*—the final stage of multi-infarct dementia, i.e. rigidity with dementia (this has gradually been accepted by most neurologists as a cause of Parkinsonism). The gait is shuffling (*marche à petits pas*) but without the forward shift of the center of gravity seen in PD, sometimes referred to as 'lower body Parkinsonism'.

Parkinsonism often responds badly to standard PD treatments and the patient's condition may sometimes be worsened by such interventions, increased confusion and falls secondary to postural hypotension being the most likely problems.

Conditions allied to Parkinson's disease

Benign essential tremor

Sometimes known as senile tremor. It can be mistaken for the pill-rolling tremor of PD but other Parkinsonian features are absent. It may be familial in some cases. It is usually present at rest and worsened by stress. It may respond to small doses of alcohol or beta-blockers.

Restless legs syndrome (Ekbom's syndrome)

This is characterized by a profound desire to move the legs and motor restlessness, which is worse at night. No drugs are licensed but levodopa or dopamine agonists before bed may be helpful.

DRUG MANAGEMENT OF PARKINSON'S DISEASE

Mechanism	Name	Prescription tips (see BNF section 4.9)
Replenish striatal dopamine	Levodopa with peripheral dopa-decarboxylase inhibitor as Sinemet® (co-careldopa) or Madopar® (co-beneldopa)	Start low, increase slowly balancing response with side-effects, with meals initially to reduce nausea, later before meals as drug competes for absorption with amino acids from a protein meal. Can use slow-release preparation from the start or to cover the night, dispersible preparation if swallowing a problem. About 85% of patients respond to levodopa
Catechol-O-methyltransferase inhibitor	Entacapone	With levodopa to reduce end of dose deterioration. May colour the urine red
Monoamine-oxidase-B inhibitor	Selegiline	With levodopa to reduce end of dose deterioration. Early monotherapy may delay need for levodopa. Some concerns about increase in mortality, sub-lingual preparation alters metabolism by avoiding first-pass and may reduce problems. Give in the morning since a mild stimulant. Avoid if orthostatic hypotension, falls or confusion and peptic ulceration
Dopamine agonists	All need very gradual dose escalation as hypotensive reactions can occur in the first few days. The therapeutic effect is mediated via the D2 receptor: their other effects depend partly on their activity at other dopaminergic receptors and whether they are derived from ergot. May be neuroprotective	
	Ergoline family • Bromocriptine • Lisuride • Pergolide • Cabergoline	Bromocriptine was the first available but is little used in the elderly due to side-effects. Lisuride and pergolide can be used alone or with levodopa. Cabergoline is the longest acting, but is not licensed for monotherapy. All rarely cause retroperitoneal fibrosis
	Non-ergoline • Ropinerole • Pramipexole • Apomorphine	Ropinerole is licensed for monotherapy or with levodopa, pramipexole as an adjunct to levodopa. Both have been associated with severe sleepiness when driving. Apomorphine is unique because, as it can only be used subcutaneously, it is given via a pen or pump under specialist supervision for intractable fluctuations
Antimuscarinic drugs	E.g. Orphenadrine and benzhexol disturbance	Little to choose between drugs, can improve drooling. Major risks in the elderly: worsening cognition, GI side-effects and urine retention

NB: If nausea is a problem, give domperidone. If a neuroleptic is needed, clozapine appears best but has restricted prescription. Olanzapine or quetiapine were thought to be better than older agents, but it may not be. Whenever any other dopaminergic agent is added to levodopa, reduce the dose of levodopa. If a PD patient is nil by mouth for any reason other than 'gut failure' put down a nasogastric tube to keep giving him/her the drugs.

Table 8.1

Progressive supranuclear palsy or Steele–Richardson–Olszewski syndrome

Extrapyramidal rigidity is of rapid onset, with paralysis of eye movement (initially upward gaze but not specific until other eye movements are involved). There is marked instability and frequent falls, pseudobulbar swallowing and speech difficulties and dementia.

Dementia of the Lewy body type

A syndrome in which Parkinsonism overlaps with features of Alzheimer's disease (AD) and psychiatric phenomena (see Chapter 4). Brain pathology shows Lewy bodies identical to those in PD but scattered throughout the cortex.

Multiple system atrophy, formerly Shy–Drager syndrome

Rigidity, with marked postural hypotension and other features of autonomic nervous system failure. Apart from attempts to maintain postural BP, there is little else in the way of intervention.

Motor-neuron disease

A degenerative condition of unknown aetiology which may easily be overlooked in elderly patients, where the UMN lesions may be assumed to be due to vascular disease. However, in motor-neuron disease, mentation usually remains normal and sensory changes are absent. The finding of LMN signs (especially muscle fibrillation) in conjunction with UMN signs is the most frequent clue to the diagnosis.

Patients with predominantly distal signs affecting legs and mobility often do well and there is only slow progression of their disease. Patients with an otherwise good quality of life and the form of the disease known as amyotrophic lateral sclerosis (mixed UMN/LMN) can be referred to a specialist neurologist for consideration of riluzole (a glutamate release inhibitor). This decreases firing of the motor neurons and prolongs the time to ventilation but is of limited benefit at any age.

Those with a bulbar presentation fare much less well, especially with the onset of speech and swallowing problems, of which the patient is only too aware. Such patients should be considered for percutaneous endoscopic gastrostomy to maintain nutrition and perhaps reduce aspiration pneumonia. The patient will normally be able to be fully involved in deciding on such a course of management.

Epilepsy in old age

After middle age, the incidence of epilepsy rises and exceeds that in children (children and adolescents up to 100/100 000 a year; aged 30–55 about 30/100 000; rising to 150/100 000 aged over 70 years).

Most fits in old age are secondary to cerebrovascular disease, i.e. up to 50%, only about 10% being due to space-occupying lesions. Other causes are sepsis, pyrexia, biochemical disturbance and drugs or alcohol (excess or withdrawal). Fits may occur in the later stages of degenerative disorders of the brain, e.g. AD.

Fits occurring in old age are usually partial seizures with a single focus of activity due to scar tissue following a stroke and may be simple partial (no impairment of consciousness), complex partial (in which consciousness is impaired) or a partial seizure, which proceeds to a generalized fit or generalized tonic clonic seizures.

Status epilepticus (SE) is a medical emergency with significant morbidity and mortality (>80 years mortality of at least 50%). The most widely accepted definition of SE is more than 30 min of either continuous seizure activity, or intermittent seizures without full recovery of consciousness between seizures. SE has a twofold increased incidence in the elderly and co-morbidity may complicate therapy and worsen prognosis. Acute or remote stroke is the most common aetiology. Non-convulsive SE (NCSE) has a wide range of clinical presentations, ranging from confusion to obtundation. It occurs commonly in elderly patients who are critically ill and in the setting of coma. EEG is the only reliable method of diagnosing NCSE. The goal of treatment for SE is to stop the fits activity as soon as possible. Usual treatment is intravenous benzodiazepine, followed by phenytoin but if treatment fails refer to intensive care for consideration of a general anaesthetic agent.

Fits may result in injury such as fractures because of underlying osteoporosis, and recovery may be prolonged by postictal symptoms and signs of weakness lasting for up to 24 h (Todd's paresis). The psychological and social consequences are at least as great as in younger patients.

Management

Investigate and, as in younger subjects, usually only treat after the second episode. Care is needed with anticonvulsants; monotherapy is preferred, especially as elderly patients are more susceptible to adverse effects (including cognitive impairment and ataxia). Carbamazepine or sodium valproate are the first-line drugs. Check the rest of the patient's medication, both because some drugs increase the chances of a fit and anti-epilepsy drugs have many interactions. Ciprofloxacin is not the best antibiotic in a post-fit chest infection because it is epileptogenic and care is needed with antidepressants. Think about safety at home—open fires should be guarded. Check whether advice on driving is relevant—do not assume that your patient is a non-driver.

Infective diseases of the central nervous system

Meningitis

Less than 10% of cases, but over 50% of deaths occur in the elderly. Problems arise because of delay in diagnosis; the symptoms are more vague in the elderly and signs, especially neck stiffness, are difficult to interpret because of the frequency of cervical spondylosis. Examination of the CSF is essential, but only perform a lumbar puncture after CT, when such facilities are available (papilloedema is frequently absent in elderly patients with raised intracranial pressure and fundoscopy is often difficult because of eye pathology).

The pnemococcus and listeria are common in old age and other atypical organisms must always be considered, especially in the very frail, malnourished and immunosuppressed. In the white population in the UK, tuberculous meningitis is more common in the elderly than in the middle aged. Cefotaxime is the appropriate empirical treatment until culture or PCR results are available.

Encephalitis

Headache, fever and malaise are followed by focal signs, fits and coma. Herpes simplex and zoster (particularly when a cranial dermatome is involved in shingles) are the most common causes. Consider the possibility early, as acyclovir is most effective when used without delay. EEG is helpful if it shows focal abnormalities particularly in the temporal lobes.

Guillain–Barré syndrome

This often occurs 1–3 weeks after a viral infection and usually takes the form of a rapidly ascending polyneuropathy. Motor features (flaccid paralysis with reduced reflexes) dominate but there may be some sensory involvement. Treatment consists of support, consider intravenous immunoglobulin or, less commonly now, plasma exchange and ventilation if respiratory muscles are involved.

Poliomyelitis

New cases are very rare in the UK because of the polio vaccination programme but you will see older people with the sequelae—usually a flaccid wasted weak leg with absent reflexes (pathology is damage to the anterior horn cells). If the damage occurred in the teens or younger the limb may be small and a caliper is often worn for foot drop.

Herpes zoster

Herpes zoster (shingles) is a reactivation of the varicella virus which has lain dormant in the dorsal root ganglia since an earlier attack of chicken pox. It follows that patients do not catch shingles from other people with varicella or shingles but that a susceptible person can catch chicken pox from someone with active shingles. Patients with shingles are often isolated in hospital to protect the nurses. It is particularly likely to afflict the debilitated and the immunosupressed and may involve a dermatome where there is spinal disease.

Clinical features
• Pain in the distribution of the dorsal root with paraesthesiae and hyperaesthesia usually precedes the rash by a couple of days, although the illness may be painless.
• The characteristic rash, like that of varicella, follows the sequence: papules—vesicles—pustules—crusts, and then ceases to be infectious. The dermatome affected is thoracic in over 50% but is trigeminal in 10–15% and, less commonly, the geniculate ganglion (Ramsay–Hunt syndrome).
• Anteriorly, the rash does not cross the mid-line, but posteriorly it follows the posterior primary ramus a few centimetres across the spinous processes. Sometimes more than one adjacent dermatome is involved but it is very seldom bilateral
• Less common features and complications include muscle wasting in the relevant segment, an internal rash in the same segment (e.g. the bladder), a mixed varicella–zoster eruption, meningoencephalitis, eye involvement and post-herpetic neuralgia.

Management
Attention to hydration and general health, plus aciclovir 800 mg five times daily by mouth or, particularly in the immunocompromised, intravenously, in the weakly evidence-based hope of minimizing the likelihood of post-herpetic neuralgia. Famciclovir can be given thrice daily. The pain may be severe and appropriate analgesia should be given.

Ophthalmic zoster
This requires urgent ophthalmological referral in case of corneal ulceration and with a view to local atropine, idoxuridine and/or aciclovir.

Post-herpetic neuralgia
Continued burning neuropathic pain over a period of months or years is said to afflict more than half of elderly patients following an attack of shingles. It is commonly severe, debilitating,

and intractable. This type of pain may respond better to tricyclic antidepressants, anticonvulsants, such as gabapentin or sodium valproate, or the application of capsaicin than to conventional analgesics.

Malignant disease
Intracranial neoplasms
Metastases are more common than cerebral primaries. In 50% of cases cerebral metastases are solitary. Primary lesions may be amenable to surgery or chemotherapy, depending on site and nature—advice will be needed from neurosurgeons and oncologists.

Cerebral metastases are most commonly from lung or breast. Palliative treatment with dexamethasone will often be beneficial in both untreatable primaries and secondaries. The window of symptom relief will be of value to both the patient and their families and help them to come to terms with the prognosis.

Non-metastatic disease of the central nervous system
This is also important in older patients and may take the form of:
1 Cerebellar syndrome.
2 Peripheral neuropathy.
3 Myasthenic syndrome.

Deficiency/toxicity states
The B group of vitamins has an important role in maintaining neurological integrity—deficiencies can have central effects, e.g. dementia, and peripheral effects, e.g. neuropathy. Neurological complications may arise before other systems are affected, e.g. sub-acute combined degeneration of the cord may precede a macrocytic anaemia. In B_{12} deficiency the findings depend on whether the spinal cord degeneration (pyramidal tracts and dorsal columns 'combined') or neuropathy dominate.

Always consider deficiency states (including myxoedema) which can usually be fairly easily confirmed and, more importantly, treated. Toxicity and deficiencies may occur together, as in alcoholic abuse. The alcohol can have a direct toxic effect on the nervous system (central and peripheral) and also lead to nutritional deficiencies because of the associated malnutrition and poor intake of nutrients, such as folate.

Diabetes can also be included in this section, as a cause of peripheral neuropathy, either symmetrical or in the form of mononeuritis multiplex.

Drugs should also be included as a cause for many neurological conditions, e.g.:
• Parkinson's disease — secondary to neuroleptics.
• Ataxia — secondary to anticonvulsant toxicity.
• Tardive dyskinesia — secondary to neuroleptics.
• Peripheral neuropathy.
• Fits.

Previous surgery may also be important, e.g. thyroidectomy, gastrectomy or ileal resection, the latter two leading to potential B_{12} malabsorption.

Entrapment neuropathies
Carpal tunnel syndrome
This can be mistaken for a peripheral neuropathy, as patients may complain of paraesthesia or dropping things but it is due to compression of the median nerve in the wrist. Look for reduced sensation over the lateral palm splitting the ring finger, wasting of the thenar eminence and weakness of abductor pollicis brevis. Steroid injections may give temporary relief but if there are signs of nerve damage refer for EMG and then surgery.

Meralgia paraesthetica
This is not serious but, if you recognize it, the patient will be grateful for the reassurance! It is

entrapment of the lateral cutaneous nerve of the thigh under inguinal ligament, commonly in the obese, resulting in numbness and tingling in the anterolateral thigh.

Further information

Bhatia, K., Brooks, D.J. & Burn, D.J et al. (2001) Updated guidelines for the management of Parkinson's disease [Parkinson's Disease Consensus Working Group]. Hospital Medicine 62(8), 456–70.
British Epilepsy Association website — Epilepsy Action: www.epilepsy.org.uk
Esmonde, T. & Cooke, S. (2002) Shunting for Normal Pressure Hydrocephalus (NPH) (Cochrane Review). The Cochrane Library, Issue 3. Update Software Ltd, Oxford.
National Institute of Neurological Disorders and Stroke website — a fantastic website with patient-friendly (hence student-friendly) material on a whole variety of neurological diseases you didn't know existed as well as the standard topics: www.ninds.nih.gov/
National Institute of Neurological Disorders and Stroke website — an example, from the website above, about Q10 and PD: http://www.ninds.nih.gov/news_and_events/pressrelease_parkinsons_coenzymeq10–101402.htm
Parkinson's Disease Society website gives excellent, up-to-date general information: www.parkinsons.org.uk
Shulman, L.M., Minager, A., Rabinstein, A. & Weiner, W.J. (2000) The use of dopamine agonists in very elderly patients with Parkinson's disease. Movement Disorders 15(4), 664–8.
Waterhouse, E.J. & DeLorenzo, R.J. (2001) Status epilepticus in older patients: epidemiology and treatment options Drugs & Aging 18(2), 133–42.
Voltz, R. (2002) Paraneoplastic neurological syndromes. Lancet Neurology 1(5), 294–305.

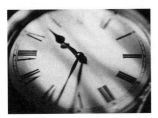

Cardiovascular Disorders

Age changes

1 Reduction in the number of cardiac myocytes secondary to apoptosis, and hypertrophy of the remainder.
2 Accumulation of intracellular lipofuscin and extracellular amyloid.
3 Increased intercellular collagen, with reduction in left ventricular (LV) diastolic compliance.
4 Patchy fibrosis of conduction system and reduction in number of pacemaker cells in sinoatrial node.
5 Reduction in adrenergic receptors.
6 Variable decline in stroke volume, cardiac output, maximum heart rate and maximal oxygen consumption. Many of these changes can be reversed by regular exercise (for the average 70–75-year-old female in the UK, walking at 5 km/h represents maximal aerobic exercise).
7 Lateral displacement of apex beat is a common finding and the cardiothoracic ratio on X-ray is greater than 50% in 70% of women aged over 70, partly owing to chest distortion, due, for example, to kyphoscoliosis.
8 Calcification of aortic-valve cusps and mitral ring.
9 Dilated, elongated aorta and stiff vessel walls due to fragmentation of elastin: afterload on ventricle rises.

Heart disease

Types seen in old age
• Ischaemic.

• Hypertensive.
• Valvular.
• Pulmonary.
• Cardiomyopathy.
• Thyrotoxic.
• Conducting-tissue disease.
• Congenital.

Manifestations
See Fig. 9.1.

Ischaemic heart disease
This is the most common cause of death in the UK and the USA. Over 80% of all deaths in the UK occur in those aged over 65. The sex incidence is equal, unlike in younger age groups. See Table 7.2, p. 58.

Presentation
• Angina.
• Acute coronary syndromes: unstable angina and MI.
• Sudden death.
• Heart failure.
• Arrhythmias.

Stable angina
• Classical retrosternal pain radiating to the left arm and throat on exertion.
• May present as breathlessness on exertion.

Management
• Reduce all risk factors (smoking, anaemia, aortic-valve disease, hypertension).
• Aspirin.

MANIFESTATIONS OF HEART DISEASE

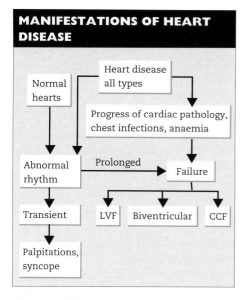

Fig. 9.1 Manifestations of heart disease.

- Advise patient to take GTN prior to exercise.
- Nitrates (ensure nitrate-free period by giving isosorbide mononitrate modified release once daily, or advice to take patch off at night).
- Beta-blockers, e.g. atenolol, unless contraindicated.
- Calcium antagonists, e.g. diltiazem.
- Nicorandil, a potassium channel opener, is a good choice for patients with low BP.

Acute coronary syndromes
Definition
The acute coronary syndromes encompass two groups: unstable angina and non-Q wave infarcts, and ST-elevation infarcts. This is because they are managed differently and they have different prognosis.

Unstable angina (and non-Q wave infarct)
1 Chest pain at rest or minimal exertion.
2 Crescendo angina on chronic background.
3 Angina of new onset on minimal exertion.

Management
- Admit to a monitored bed if possible.

- Bed rest.
- Aspirin.
- Glyceryl trinitrate spray/tablet.
- Intravenous glyceryl trinitrate or buccal nitrate.
- LMWH.
- Beta-blockers (atenolol or metoprolol), unless contraindicated.
- If not settling, add calcium antagonist (diltiazem).
- The use of intravenous glcyoprotein IIa/IIIb blockers (e.g. tirofiban and abciximab which prevent platelets from cross-linking and therefore prevent platelet aggregation) has not been established in older people.
- Caution — watch for bradycardia and hypotension.
- If still not settling, urgent angiography with a view to revascularization, e.g. PTCA or CABG.
- Following successful management, reduce all possible risk factors and establish oral regime.

ST-elevation myocardial infarction
Increasing evidence shows that older people with acute MI respond just as well to thrombolysis as younger patients. However, several factors militate against this: atypical presentations (see 'Presenting clinical features of myocardial infarction' box, p. 79), late presentation to hospital, increased incidence of non-Q wave infarcts which do not respond to thrombolysis, non-diagnostic ECGs because of left bundle branch block, etc. and the multiplicity of co-morbidities and contraindications. If the diagnostic criteria are met, the management should not be significantly different from that of younger patients.

Management
- Give oxygen and opiates whilst diagnosis being confirmed.
- Stat. dose of aspirin, to be continued on daily basis if no contraindication.
- Admit to monitored bed.
- In the case of infarction with ST-elevation, thrombolyse with intravenous streptokinase.

Presenting clinical features of myocardial infarction

- 'Typical' chest pain (20%)
- Sudden death
- Mild chest discomfort, sometimes attributed to indigestion
- Abdominal pain
- 'Silent', i.e. ECG changes or rise in MB fraction of creatine kinase (CKMB) or troponin levels with no chest pain (up to 45% in the longitudinal Framingham Heart study), found in a patient admitted after a fall, or 'off legs'.
- Heart failure, shortness of breath.
- Arrhythmias.
- Functional decline, or confusion.
- A fall, found lying on floor unconscious, hypotension.
- Stroke.
- Peripheral gangrene.
- Post-operative fever, tachycardia, hypotension.

There is evidence that there is increased risk of intracerebral haemorrhage with tissue plasminogen activator (tPA) in older people.
- Oxygen.
- LMWH
- Treatment with oral beta-blockers, again to be continued if no contraindications, has been proven to be of benefit to older people.
- ACE inhibitors in patients with evidence of LV failure (to reduce LV re-modelling).
- Consider whether cholesterol-lowering treatment is indicated.
- Older people should have equal access to cardiac rehabilitation facilities post-MI.
- Consider whether exercise or pharmacological stress testing is appropriate if the patient is biologically fit.

Heart failure

Heart failure is an extremely common cause of hospital admissions, re-admissions, reduced function and institutionalization. Although often biventricular, it is conventionally divided into congestive cardiac failure and acute LV failure.

Acute left ventricular failure
Clinical features
- Severe breathlessness, orthopnoea, paroxysmal nocturnal dyspnoea.
- Frothy pink sputum.
- On examination, there may be tachycardia, a third heart sound, crackles at the lung bases and, sometimes, pleural effusions.

Management
- The patient is likely to be sat bolt upright already.
- Give oxygen via a face mask.
- Urinary catheter to monitor urine output.
- GTN infusion to off-load right heart and reduce angina if present. Aim to keep systolic BP above 90 mmHg.
- Intravenous loop diuretics.
- Opiates are very useful in this situation, as they not only reduce anxiety and pain therefore reducing oxygen demand, but they also reduce pre-load.
- Treat precipitant, e.g. fast AF.
- Exclude acute MI.
- Treat co-existing pneumonia with intravenous antibiotics.
- Consider short-term treatment with an intravenous inotrope, e.g. dobutamine, if the patient is normally very fit and independent.

Congestive cardiac failure
Prevalence
In people aged over 65, ranges from 5–10%, with annual mortality 10–50%, depending on severity. Frequent features include fatigue, functional decline, confusion, falls and cachexia.

NB: Ankle oedema is often non-cardiac — e.g. chair-bound immobility increases venous pressure, due to gravity, loss of muscle-pump activity and pressure on thigh veins by the chair.

Causes of biventricular heart failure
- Ischaemic heart disease.
- Hypertension.

- Valvular heart disease.
- Cor pulmonale including pulmonary emboli.
- Thyrotoxicosis.
- Severe anaemia.
- Arrhythmias, especially fast AF.
- Drugs, including NSAIDs.
- Cardiomyopthies.

Treatment
1 Advise the patient to reduce salt and fluid intake.
2 Stop smoking.
3 Control the rhythm.
4 Diuretics to reduce overload.
5 ACE inhibitor, unless contraindicated by poor renal function, hypotension or aortic-valve disease (initiate in hospital in high-risk cases). If not tolerated, hydralazine or a nitrate should be tried.
6 Angiotensin II blockers can be used in patients who cannot tolerate ACE inhibitors.
7 Increase diuretics and ACE inhibitors as required/tolerated.
8 There is an increasing role for beta-blockers such as carvedilol and bisoprolol. They are now indicated for most grades of heart failure. They should be started at very low doses and titrated up as tolerated.
9 There is now evidence that spironolactone reduces morbidity and mortality in heart failure, and is often well-tolerated in older people.
10 Treat causative or precipitating factors, e.g. valve surgery, if indicated, hypertension, anaemia.
11 Digoxin for its positive inotropic effect in sinus-rhythm is probably useful in severe disease.
12 Anticoagulation is only indicated if there is a risk of thromboembolic disease.
13 Add metolazone to diuretic regime for massive oedema.
14 Terminal stage—opiates, oxygen as required.

Diastolic dysfunction
Upward shift of pressure–volume relationship so that the normal LV volume and ventricular diastolic pressure is elevated. This pressure is transmitted back to the RA and pulmonary veins causing pulmonary congestion.

Think of it where there is a history of hypertension and the heart size is normal, and in patients with diabetes and infiltrative cardiomyopthies such as amyloidosis.

Current advice is that off-loading with diuretics is detrimental; try low-salt diet. Avoid digoxin.

Hypertension
Definition
Traditionally, sustained readings on separate occasions greater than 130/85 according to WHO-ISH hypertension guidelines committee. Isolated systolic hypertension implies only systolic pressure elevated (above 130).

Prevalence
Among people aged 65–74, ranges from 45% to 64% according to different surveys.

Effects of hypertension
Major risk factor for atherosclerosis and thus stroke, coronary-artery disease and peripheral vascular disease.

Effects of treatment
Up to age 80, treatment produces considerable benefit (more than in younger subjects) in total mortality and cardiovascular morbidity and mortality—but sometimes at the expense of making the patient feel worse. After age 80 there is as yet insufficient evidence to support urging treatment on all patients.

Treatment
1 Low-salt, low-calorie, low-alcohol, high-exercise regime.
2 Drugs:
   (a) Thiazide diuretics.
   (b) Beta-blockers.
   (c) Calcium antagonists.
   (d) ACE inhibitors.

Aim
Probably a level of not greater than 140/90.

Atrial fibrillation
Prevalence is about 5–10% in people over age of 75. The incidence increases markedly in those with biventricular heart disease and valvular heart disease.

Most common causes
• Ischaemic heart disease • CCF • Valvular heart disease • Hypertension • Thyroid disease • PE • Pneumonia

Consequences
1 Reduction in cardiac output causes fatigue, lethargy, reduced exercise tolerance, heart failure.
2 Slow AF (due to digoxin or to conducting-tissue disease) may be associated with pauses. If only at night, these are not usually significant, but if symptomatic, may require pacing.
3 Systemic emboli, mainly to brain (stroke risk is increased by five times) and lower limbs.

Treatment
1 Acute onset, under 48 h:

(a) Admit and give LMWH.
(b) May revert spontaneously, especially if due to pneumonia or MI.
If persisting beyond 48 h, consider cardioversion, using direct-current (DC) shock or intravenous flecainide, or amiodarone acutely or after 1 month's anticoagulation (to be continued for a further 1 month afterwards, together with maintenance sotalol or amiodarone to prevent recurrence).
2 Consider sotalol or amiodarone to maintain sinus rhythm.
3 Otherwise, control heart rate—aim at 90 b.p.m. Digitalization orally is standard therapy but verapamil *or* a beta-blocker in addition will be faster and more effective; amiodarone orally or intravenously (but central line usually recommended) also effective and sometimes restores sinus rhythm.
4 Exclude correctable causes—thyrotoxicosis and (possibly) valvular disease.
5 For AF of comparatively recent origin (1 year) without serious heart disease on echocardiography, which would make recurrence almost inevitable, consider referral for possible elective cardioversion.
6 It is important to consider anticoagulation for those remaining in AF. The risk of stroke associated with AF in the context of rheumatic heart disease is increased 17-fold and 2–7-fold in non-rheumatic heart disease.
7 Paroxysmal AF: digoxin is potentially harmful; sotalol or amiodarone reduce frequency of attacks and ventricular rate during them. Low stroke risk: give aspirin.

Indications for aspirin vs. warfarin	
Aspirin 300 mg/day • Frequent changes of medication • Dementia • Tendency to fall • Uncontrolled hypertension • Consider clopidogrel for those intolerant of aspirin	**Warfarin INR 2–3** • Previous stroke • Mitral-valve disease • Enlarged left atrium • Poor LV function • Controlled hypertension

Valvular heart disease

Systolic murmurs are audible in 30–60% of elderly patients and when significant arise from the mitral valve in 50%, the aortic valve in 25% and both in 25% of cases.

Mitral regurgitation

This condition is thought to be associated with some cases of transient cerebral or retinal ischaemia.

The commonest causes of mitral regurgitation in elderly people

- Calcification of mitral ring
- Dilatation of left ventricle and mitral ring
- Mucoid (myxomatous) degeneration of cusps
- Floppy mitral valve with prolapse of posterior cusp
- Papillary-muscle dysfunction—usually ischaemic
- Rupture of chordae tendineae (often partial)
- Infective endocarditis
- Rheumatic heart disease

Calcific aortic stenosis

The triad of symptoms is angina, breathlessness and syncope or presyncope. The murmur may be unimpressive but an echocardiogram will give the gradient across the valve and, if over 60 mm, this should prompt consideration of surgery.

Infective endocarditis

- The mortality remains 15–30%, with about 200 deaths in England and Wales each year.
- The majority of cases are now patients aged 60 or over.
- Previously unrecognized calcific valve disease is the major risk factor in Western countries.
- Dental and genitourinary procedures should be covered with prophylactic antibiotics, although it is not clear which other invasive activities should be covered.
- Patients with prosthetic heart valves require scrupulous prophylaxis for even trivial procedures.

Clinical features

The diagnosis depends on clinical criteria; it must be excluded in patients presenting with:
- Chronic fever.
- Weight-loss.
- Malaise.
- Intermittent confusion.
- New or changing murmurs help clinch the diagnosis but absence of a murmur does not exclude it.
- 'Classic signs' such as Janeway lesions and Osler's nodes are rare.

Investigations

- Raised ESR and CRP.
- Mild-moderate normocytic normochromic anaemia.
- Three sets of blood should be taken at least an hour apart from different sites. *Streptococcus viridans* is the commonest organism.
- Urine dipstix may show haematuria and or proteinuria.
- Transthoracic echocardiography.
- Proceed to transoesophageal echocardiography (TOE) if transthoracic echocardiography is negative and the clinical suspicion is high.

Management

- Intravenous antibiotics as guided by the microbiology department for the first 2 weeks.
- Oral antibiotics for a further 2–4 weeks.
- If the valve is badly damaged, the organism is resistant or if the patient is in refractory heart failure, the valve may need replacement.
- Advise the patient about the need for antibiotic prophylaxis for procedures in the future.

Orthostatic (postural) hypotension

Any fall in BP on standing up is poorly tolerated in older people because cerebral autoregulation is often defective, especially in hypertensive subjects. The current definition is a fall of 20 mm or more in systolic BP or 10 mm diastolic BP (prevalence 20–30% of community-living elderly people). It may be an incidental finding, unless good correlation with symptoms and with distress caused by standing up. Symptoms include dizziness, presyncope, syncope, falls and visual disturbances.

Causes

- Hypovolaemia due to salt and water depletion
- Autonomic nervous system dysfunction (Chapter 12)
- Drugs—antihypertensives, including diuretics, phenothiazines, antidepressants, levodopa, vasodilators (including alcohol), narcotic analgesics, verapamil, disopyramide
- Prolonged recumbency
- Cardiac disease (e.g. infarction)
- Varicose veins
- Addison's disease

Investigations

- Repeated measurement of postural BP, especially in the morning and after meals.
- Twenty-four hour BP monitoring.
- Urea and electrolytes.
- Short Synacthen test.

Treatment

- Correct cause if identified.
- Advice concerning sensible precautions ('have a bath with a friend').
- Compression hosiery—full-length, preferably tights.
- Medication—fludrocortisone, or midodrine, a peripheral alpha agonist.
- Head-up tilt to bed (20°) to reduce nocturnal natriuresis.

Syncope, presyncope, faints, funny turns

- This possibility should be considered in patients with recurrent falls.
- There may be a history of a blackout.
- However, some patients with syncope have amnesia for the blackout.
- Cerebral blood flow is about 50 mL/100 g/min in older people but is lower in those with hypertension or atherosclerosis.
- Symptoms of cerebral ischaemia occur when the blood flow is reduced to 25–30 mL/100 g/min.
- Differential diagnosis is from epilepsy (Fig. 9.2): cerebral anoxia readily causes seizures and some forms of epilepsy are difficult to distinguish from syncope but are usually followed by post-ictal confusion lasting more than 20 min.

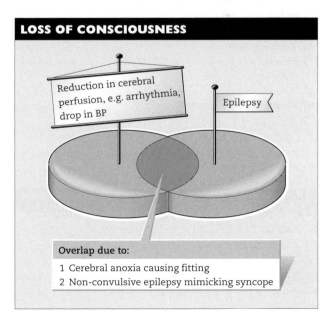

LOSS OF CONSCIOUSNESS

Reduction in cerebral perfusion, e.g. arrhythmia, drop in BP

Epilepsy

Overlap due to:
1 Cerebral anoxia causing fitting
2 Non-convulsive epilepsy mimicking syncope

Fig. 9.2 Transient loss of consciousness.

Causes of a single episode
- MI.
- PE.
- GI bleed.

Causes of recurrent episodes (Table 9.1)
- Disturbance of heart rhythm.
- Hypotension (Table 9.2).
- Aortic stenosis.
- Carotid sinus hypersensitivity, three sub-types:
    (a) Cardioinhibitory, carotid sinus massage (CSM) produces a pause longer than 3 s in duration.
    (b) Vasodepressor type: CSM produces a fall in systolic BP of >50 mmHg in the absence of bradycardia.
    (c) Mixed subtype.

Carotid sinus massage
- The patient is lying down with their head in a neutral position.
- The carotid sinus is massaged longitudinally for 5 s on each side separately, allowing 30 s between.
- Contraindications: recent MI, ventricular tachycardia.
- If there is a suspicion of carotid disease, this should be excluded by carotid doppler before starting.

Indications for pacemaker
1 Stokes–Adams attacks are an indication for urgent pacing.
2 Persistent failure, lethargy and poor exercise tolerance are indications for pacing in patients with atrioventricular (AV) block.
3 In the absence of these indications, practice varies from pacing all patients with complete heart block to selecting those with a ventricular rate below 40. This includes AF with partial block and a slow ventricular response.
4 Sinus-node disease with bradycardia or pauses over 3 s, with the brady–tachy syn-

---

RECURRENT FUNNY TURNS

History — patient (palpitations?) and witness (fitting?)
Examination — includes lying and standing BP, heart rhythm, aortic ejection murmur, ECG with rhythm strip and gentle carotid massage, unless bruit, history of ventricular tachycardia, recent stroke or MI
1 Palpitations/abrupt syncope/abnormal ECG → Holter monitor
2 Angina, systolic murmur → echo
3 Aura, postictal state → EEG
4 Light-headed → ambulatory BP monitor
5 Refer cardiology for sophisticated monitoring
6 ?Tilt table at 70° 20–60 min

Table 9.1 Elucidation of recurrent funny turns.

HYPOTENSION CAUSES

Postural
Post-prandial
Exertional
Carotid-sinus sensitivity (bradycardia ± hypotension)
Malignant vasovagal syndrome (vasodepressor type)

Table 9.2 Causes of recurrent hypotension.

drome, with AV block or with 'chronotropic incompetence' (a failure to speed up to cope with exercise—elderly people are unable to compensate for this with a rise in the stroke volume).

5 Carotid-sinus sensitivity with recurrent syncope.

Vascular disease

Abdominal aortic aneurysm

Affects 3% of people aged over 50 and causes 6000–10000 deaths annually in England and Wales. Up to 4 cm, regular ultrasound screening; over 5.0–5.5 cm, advise surgery if patient suitable. Unoperated—5% rupture per annum if diameter 5–6 cm, rising exponentially if larger.

Peripheral vascular disease

Presentation

1 Intermittent claudication.

2 Critical ischaemia (rest pain, ulcers, necrotic or septic skin lesions), sometimes following trauma or a haemodynamic crisis. Those of limited mobility may not give a history of previous claudication.

Diagnosis

Affected extremities may be discoloured, with trophic changes in skin and nails (hair loss sensitive but extremely non-specific), cool and pulseless, bruits over femoral, superficial femoral (frequent site of obstruction) or popliteal arteries. Elicit blanching on elevation and delayed hyperaemia and venous filling on dependency. Measure ankle systolic pressure with Doppler probe—should be 0.8 of the brachial pressure.

Management

See Fig. 9.3.

Giant-cell arteritis

The features of this disease are given below. The response to high-dose corticosteroids (initially 40–80 mg daily) is dramatic. The dose is very gradually reduced to a level of 5–10 mg,

depending on the ESR, and continued for 2 years. Protect bones from accelerated osteoporosis.

Features of giant-cell arteritis

- Late age of onset
- Pathology—thickening of intima, giant-cell infiltration
- Polymyalgia rheumatica (Chapter 6)
- Headache
- Scalp tenderness
- Tender, thickened superficial temporal arteries
- Constitutional—fever, weight loss
- Occlusion of short posterior ciliary artery with blindness
- Jaw claudication
- Pain in tongue
- Stroke
- Coronary artery involvement
- Peripheral arterial involvement
- Functional decline
- Anaemia, abnormal liver function tests
- High ESR

Venous and pulmonary thromboembolic disease

Diagnosis of DVT requires confirmation by ultrasound scan of thigh veins and, if negative but strongly suspected, venography. Treatment of DVT in patients who are otherwise well can now be done as an out patient with treatment doses of LMWH for at least 4 days, together with warfarin as per protocol. PE is also treated with LMWH to prevent further thrombosis and allow endogenous fibrinolysis to occur. Once the diagnosis is confirmed, start warfarin. In the case of massive PE—consider thrombolysis.

Prevention is always preferable to cure: consider compression stockings and prophylactic doses of low-molecular-weight subcutaneous

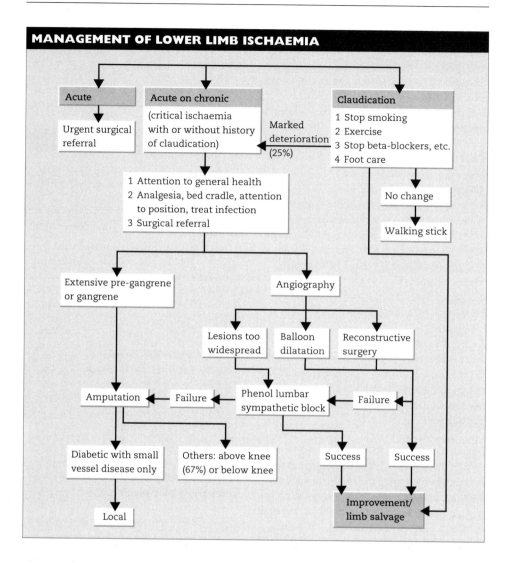

Fig. 9.3 Management of lower limb ischaemia.

heparin in high-risk hospitalized patients, such as those with pneumonia or heart failure.

Risk factors for pulmonary embolism
• Increasing age.
• Immobility.
• Surgery especially abdominal.
• Fractures, especially lower limb.
• Malignant disease.
• Obesity.
• Procoagulant states.

Pulmonary embolism presentation

- Typical—pleuritic pain, haemoptysis (25%)
- Collapse
- Sudden death
- Fever
- Breathless attacks
- Arrhythmia
- Cough, 'pneumonia'
- Bronchospasm
- Right heart failure
- Pulmonary oedema
- Increasing exertional dyspnoea
- Confusion
- Falls
- Functional decline, hypotension

Diagnosis of pulmonary embolism

- ECG most commonly shows sinus tachycardia. Rarely there may be signs of right heart stress, or new AF.
- The CXR is often normal but may show segmental collapse, a raised hemidiaphragm or a pleural effusion.
- Blood gases may be normal early on but hypoxaemia is suggestive of PE.
- The mainstay of diagnosis is by isotope V/Q scan.
- If there is co-existent cardiorespiratory disease spiral CT is very useful.
- Pulmonary angiography is the gold standard where available.
- D-dimer: this is sensitive but not specific, so if normal helps to exclude thromboembolism.

Duration of anticoagulants

- Calf vein (post-operatively) — 6 weeks.
- Calf vein (other) — 3 months.
- Proximal vein or PE (unless identifiable cause) — 6 months.

Further information

Anon. (1993) Summary of 1993 WHO/International Society of Hypertension guidelines for the management of mild hypertension. *British Medical Journal* **307**, 1541–6.

Bennet, N. (1994) Hypertension in the elderly. *Lancet* **344**, 447–9.

Cairns, J.A. (1995) Unstable angina. *Lancet* **346**, 1644–5.

Chalmers. J. (1999) 1999 World Health Organization –International Society of Hypertension Guidelines for the Management of Hypertension. *Journal of Hypertension* **17**, 151–83.

Channer, K.S. (1996) Treatment of atrial fibrillation. *Prescribers' Journal* **36**, 146–53.

Consumers Association (1996) The antiarrhythmic treatment of atrial fibrillation. *Drug and Therapeutics Bulletin* **34**, 41–5.

Dargie, H.J. & McMurray, J.J.V. (1994) Diagnosis and management of heart failure. *British Medical Journal* **308**, 321–8.

Insua, J.T., Sacks, H.S., Lau, T.-S et al. (1994) Drug treatment of hypertension in the elderly: a meta-analysis. *Annals of Internal Medicine* **121**, 355–62.

King, D. (1996) Diagnosis and management of heart failure in the elderly. *Postgraduate Medical Journal* **72**, 577–80.

Lip, G.Y.H. (1995 & 1996) ABC of atrial fibrillation. *British Medical Journal* **311**, 1361–3; **312**, 45–9.

McMurray, J.J.V. & Rankin, A. (1994) Treatment of congestive cardiac failure, atrial fibrillation and arrhythmia. *British Medical Journal* **309**, 1631–5.

More, R.S. & Chaubran, A. (1996) Anti-thrombotic therapy for non-rheumatic atrial fibrillation. *Quarterly Journal of Medicine* **89**, 409–14.

Morely-Davies, H. & Cobbe, S.M. (1997) Cardiac pacing. *Lancet* **349**, 41–6.

Mulrow, C.D., Cornell, J.A., Herrera, C.R., Kadri, A., Farnett, L. & Aguilar, C. (1994) Hypertension in the elderly. *Journal of the American Medical Association* **272**, 1932–8.

North of England Stable Angina Guideline Development Group (1996) Summary version of evidence based on guidelines for the primary care management of stable angina. *British Medical Journal* **312**, 827–32.

Sever, P., Beevers, G., Bulpitt, C. et al. (1993) Management guidelines in essential hypertension. *British Medical Journal* **306**, 983–7.

Staessen, J.A. (1996) How far should the blood pressure be lowered? *Lancet* **348**, 696–7.

Swales, J. (1994) Pharmacological treatment of hypertension. *Lancet* **344**, 380–5.

Swannell, A.J. (1997) Polymyalgia rheumatica and temporal arteritis: diagnosis and management. *British Medical Journal* **314**, 1329–32.

Van der Vliet, J.A. & Boll, A.P.M. (1997) Abdominal aortic aneurysm. *Lancet* **349**, 863–5.

Wei, J.Y. (1992) Age and the cardiovascular system. *New England Journal of Medicine* **327**, 1735–9.

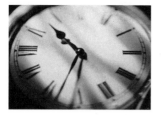

Respiratory Disease

Importance

Respiratory disease causes approximately 20% of all deaths and some 25% of hospital admissions. Death rates for respiratory disease increase steeply with age, and three-quarters of respiratory disease deaths occur among people 65 years or older. The three main killing diseases are lung cancer, pneumonia, and chronic obstructive pulmonary disease (COPD). COPD causes about 90% of respiratory disability. Most asthma deaths are among older people with two-thirds of the 1366 asthma deaths in 1998 among people aged 65 years or older. Older patients with asthma have more frequent hospital admissions.

Age changes

Physiology
Age-related changes affect virtually all aspects of the respiratory system. Structural and functional changes occur, decreasing efficiency of gas transfer. However, because the lungs have huge reserve capacity, significant clinical issues only arise when an elderly person becomes sick unless lung function has been progressively damaged by smoking or air pollution. Older people may have difficulty performing many lung function tests but simple spirometry is usually possible.

1 Reduced lung elasticity and chest-wall compliance lead to air trapping, a rise in residual volume and a fall in the forced vital capacity (FVC), forced expiratory volume in 1 s (FEV$_1$) and peak expiratory flow.

2 Increase in airway size and loss of alveolar surface decrease the lung volume available for gas exchange and increase dead space, reducing efficiency of gas exchange. Premature closure of small airways results in ventilation-perfusion mismatching, contributing to an increase in the alveolar-arterial oxygen gradient. Arterial oxygen tension (PaO$_2$) falls from 12.7 kPa at age 30 to 10 kPa at age 60.

3 Oxygen delivery to tissues (VO$_2$ max) decreases due to age-related decreases in cardiac output and body muscle mass, as well as ventilation–perfusion mismatching and decreased alveolar volume.

4 Mucociliary protection of the lower airway is impaired.

Examination
Check the rate and pattern of respiration. Tachypnoea suggests a cardio-respiratory problem and this can be very useful if the patient cannot give much history. Cheyne–Stokes respiration, in which the breathing becomes progressively shallower sometimes culminating in an apnoeic episode before becoming progressively deeper again in a cyclical pattern, is commoner in the elderly. It is often seen in stroke but may occur in apparently normal individuals.

Note the chest shape. Significant kyphosis is usually now due to osteoporosis (previously TB). The patient may forget significant surgery; thyroid and thoracotomy scars are easy to miss. The normal trachea may deviate slightly to the right around an unfolded aorta. Many older patients have basal crackles of no significance that clear on coughing. Conversely, if the patient has poor air entry an area of consolidation may appear silent. A silent chest is a danger sign in airway obstruction. After a fall, check for bruising of the chest wall and 'spring' the ribcage for fractures (pneumonia usually follows). Remember other systems associated with chest problems, e.g. aspiration in Parkinson's disease, and check for heart failure. Oxygen saturation measured by a fingertip probe is a useful bedside test. The admission CXR in an ill old patient is often difficult to interpret; usually taken AP or even supine (check for scapular lines), often with rotation (check relation of heads of clavicles to spinous processes), sometimes with the head in the chest and with poor inspiration. A subtle diagnosis may require a repeat film when the patient is improving.

Upper respiratory tract infection

Rhinoviruses (mostly picornaviruses) cause coryza, the common cold. This is a mild systemic upset with nasal symptoms, but older people, particularly smokers and those with pre-existing chronic illness may develop lower-respiratory complications.

Influenza is usually debilitating in the elderly, particularly in the presence of chronic heart, chest or renal disease, or diabetes and may be complicated by pneumonia, especially due to *Staphylococcus aureus*. Everyone aged over 65 years should be offered immunization in October/November. The influenza viruses are constantly altering their antigenic structure, so every year the WHO recommends which strains should be included in the 'flu vaccine. The vaccine may cause a mild local reaction and hypersensitivity to egg products is a contraindication. Immunity takes 2–4 weeks to develop and lasts 6–8 months. There is evidence that immunization of staff is the best way to protect residents of institutions and some hospitals offer free vaccination to their staff.

Acute breathlessness

The acutely dyspnoeic elderly patient is a very common medical emergency.

Common causes of acute respiratory distress

- LV failure
- Pneumonia
- Exacerbation of COPD
- Exacerbation of asthma
- Pulmonary embolism
- Pneumothorax
- Inhaled foreign body (stridor, choking)

Airway obstruction

Most cases are due to COPD but a number of patients have long-standing asthma and late-onset asthma may be increasing. COPD includes chronic bronchitis, defined clinically as sputum production on most days for 3 months of 2 successive years, and emphysema, defined histologically as air space dilatation due to destruction of their walls. There may be a reversible component to the obstruction especially in asthmatics who have smoked.

Features of severe attack of airways obstruction requiring admission

- Previous admission for same condition
- Use of domiciliary oxygen
- Patient cannot complete sentences
- Respiratory rate >25/min
- Pulse rate > 110 b.p.m. (unreliable in AF)
- Peak flow <50% of patient's normal or predicted
- $Po_2 < 8\,kPa$, $Pco_2 > 6.7\,kPa$ on air

Management of acute exacerbation of airway obstruction

1 Humidified oxygen: 24% or 28%, if CO_2 retention and check arterial blood gases (ABGs). If a patient on oxygen becomes drowsy, remove the mask, shake awake and check ABGs.

2 β_2-agonist (2.5–5 mg salbutamol) by nebulizer using humidified air not oxygen as the carrier.

3 Prednisolone 20–40 mg daily (100 mg i.v. hydrocortisone if unable to take tablets). Elderly patients may have problems with short courses of steroids including steroid psychosis, CCF precipitated by fluid overload and unmasking of diabetes (as well as the well known long-term complications).

4 Intravenous fluids.

5 Antibiotics (amoxicillin 500 mg t.d.s., clarithromycin 500 mg b.d. if penicillin allergic or if more severe, co-amoxiclav 625 mg t.d.s. initially intravenously if indicated. Treat as pneumonia (see below) if sputum purulent, patient ill or febrile, high WBC or CRP, or X-ray evidence of infection.

6 Antimuscarinic (ipratropium bromide 500 µg) by nebulizer.

7 Monitor temperature, pulse rate and respiration, oxygen saturation and peak flow.

8 Chest physiotherapy if secretions retained.

9 Consider DVT prophylaxis — enoxaparin 40 mg o.d. or thrombo-embolic device (TED) stockings.

10 Aminophylline infusion if obstruction remains severe (not if on oral theophylline unless levels are available).

11 If the patient is beginning to tire and pH < 7.35 consider:

    (a) Nasal non-invasive positive-pressure ventilation (has largely replaced doxapram and a good option in those patients who are poor candidates for intubation because it may be difficult to extubate).

    (b) Intensive care for ventilation if above measures ineffective. Find out about the patient's functional status prior to this illness before contacting ITU to discuss admission.

Post-acute/chronic phase

1 Unless the patient is very disabled, stopping smoking is still worthwhile.

2 Consider a steroid trial (30 mg Prednisolone for 2 weeks). Greater than 10% improvement in peak flow indicates element of reversibility.

3 Stabilize on maintenance regime of inhaled β_2-agonist ± muscarinic agonist (tiotropium looks promising) ± steroid, ensuring inhaler and spacer device understood by patient. Large-scale studies of combination inhaler therapy of salmeterol/fluticasone (1000 µg) b.d. or eformoterol/budesonide (800 µg) b.d. over 1 year reduce exacerbations of COPD by 25–30% in patients with moderate to severe COPD (FEV_1 < 50% predicted) but these combinations are expensive. Prescribe salbutamol or equivalent as 'rescue medication'.

4 Consider supplying antibiotics and oral steroids for patient to initiate self-treatment of an exacerbation (with clear instructions).

5 Pulmonary rehabilitation programme for those with respiratory disability (exercise and nutrition).

6 Depression is common — consider a SSRI.

7 Domiciliary oxygen can be provided for symptomatic relief (cylinder) or if the patient meets criteria listed in the BNF (PO_2 on air when stable <7.3 kPa) and will wear oxygen for at least 15 h a day, long-term oxygen therapy (LTOT) to improve life expectancy (concentrator).

8 Palliative care of end-stage chronic lung disease. In addition to oxygen, an opiate or benzodiazepine can relieve respiratory distress.

Pneumonia

The commonest organism is *Streptococcus pneumoniae* followed by *Haemophilus influenzae*, *Mycoplasma* in epidemic years (every 3rd year), viruses, *Branhamella*, *Legionella*, *Chlamydia pneumoniae* and *Staph. aureus* — especially during outbreaks of influenza. Prevalent pathogens and their sensitivities vary from one locality to another. It is often difficult to identify the organism, as elderly patients often swallow their sputum, but blood culture is sometimes positive.

Presentation may be typical or atypical, with tachypnoea and functional decline. Pre-existing airway disease is almost certain to deteriorate.

Aspiration pneumonia is common in older patients with swallowing disorders or following an episode of unconsciousness.

Features indicating life-threatening pneumonia

- Respiratory rate > 30/min
- Diastolic BP < 60 mmHg
- Arterial Po_2 < 8 kPa
- WBC > 20 000 × 10^9/L or < 4000 × 10^9/L
- Multiple lobes affected on CXR
- Confusion*
- Blood urea > 7 mmol/L*
- Serum albumin < 35 g/L*
- Co-morbidity, e.g. diabetes, heart disease

*Very common non-specific findings in sick old people—in whom all pneumonia is life-threatening

Pneumococcal pneumonia has a mortality rate approaching 35% in elderly subjects. In addition to splenectomized patients where it is mandatory, frail patients with chronic heart, lung, renal, liver disease and diabetes should be offered pneumococcal vaccine, which usually provides immunity for 5–10 years.

Antibiotics are traditionally given intravenously in the first instance to those with life-threatening features, as well as those unable to swallow, although there is little evidence of greater effectiveness by this route. The regime in adults has usually included a second-generation cephalosporin, such as cefotaxime, but many hospitals discourage cephalosporin use in older people, as they are strongly associated with the often serious (for the patient) and always disruptive (for the hospital ward) complication of *Clostridium difficile* colitis. In older people, a recommended regime for severe community-acquired pneumonia is benzylpenicillin 1.2 g q.d.s. plus ciprofloxacin 200 mg b.d. i.v., adding flucloxacillin 1 g q.d.s. after 'flu or metronidazole 500 mg i.v. t.d.s. if aspiration is suspected. Remember to reduce the dose of ciprofloxacin in renal impairment, watch the INR if anticoagu-

lated and swap to oral as soon as possible as it is very expensive intravenously and well absorbed orally. Less severe pneumonia may be treated with amoxicillin 500 mg t.d.s. and clarithromycin 500 mg b.d.

Other measures include oxygen (same precautions as in airway obstruction), intravenous fluids, physiotherapy for retained secretions and relief of bronchospasm if prominent.

Pulmonary tuberculosis

Despite repeated warnings in the international literature, the authors have yet to see a resurgence in pulmonary tuberculosis (TB) in elderly patients within their geographically and perhaps socially limited practice—even among patients on long-term steroids. Look out for the signs and X-ray findings of TB from the pre-drug era (chest deformity from thoracoplasty, scars in neck from TB node removal, phrenic crush or artificial pneumothorax, the common findings of apical calcification, granuloma and calcified lymph nodes or more rarely 'balls' on the CXR (plombage). Haemoptysis may indicate recrudescence of TB or a complication, such as the development of a fungus ball (aspergilloma) in an old cavity. Remain alert to the possibility of TB (especially in elderly immigrants from the Indian sub-continent and in conurbations especially London) and send sputum for acid-fast bacillus (AFB) and request a radiology and chest opinion if TB is possible. Infections with atypical mycobacteria occur in damaged lung and immuno-suppressed patients.

Pleural effusion

Common causes

- Heart failure
- Pneumonia—empyema often presents atypically
- Pulmonary embolism
- Malignancy (1° or 2°)—especially if 'white-out' on CXR

Effusions are classified as an exudate (protein > 30 g/L) or transudate but this can be less clear in a frail elderly patient with a low serum albumin. Unless there is obvious heart failure, when it is sensible to monitor the response to diuretics, diagnostic aspiration is usually necessary and therapeutic aspiration may be needed to relieve breathlessness from a huge effusion. Seek advice about pleurodesis in malignancy and irradiating the track to prevent seeding in mesothelioma.

Bronchiectasis

Bronchiectasis, abnormal irreversible dilatation of the muscular and elastic walls of the bronchi resulting in chronic infection, is usually post-infectious (measles, whooping cough or TB) in this age group. The features and treatment overlap with recurrent chest infections and COPD; physiotherapy and postural drainage are particularly important.

Chest trauma

- *Rib fracture* — common after mild trauma, e.g. coughing fit.
- *Diagnosis* — local tenderness and pain on springing chest.
- *Complications* — shallow breathing and reluctance to cough may cause sputum retention and segmental collapse. Pneumo- or haemothorax: refer for usual treatment.
- *Treatment* — adequate regular analgesia (e.g. paracetamol, an NSAID with gut protection or COX-2 inhibitor and meptazinol or tramadol), usually with physiotherapy; is essential to avoid infection. If associated with minor trauma, treat long-term for osteoporosis.

Carcinoma of the bronchus

This is the commonest life-threatening cancer in the West, is rapidly increasing in frequency in females and has become mainly a disease of older people (75% of cases aged over 60 in one series, 66% aged over 65 in another). The histological classification is into squamous (60%), small (oat) cell (20%), adenocarcinoma and large-cell types; adenocarcinomas are not smoking-related. Presentation may be respiratory with cough, haemoptysis, dyspnoea or slowly resolving infection (repeat CXR 6 weeks after pneumonia to check resolution) but is often late, with symptoms relating to distant spread or non-metastatic metabolic complications. Surgery offers the possibility of cure in local disease if the patient is fit enough and lung function is adequate ($FEV_1 > 1.5$ L). Lobectomy at the age of 70 has a mortality of up to 15%, and pneumonectomy 30%; the former procedure is rarely appropriate for patients aged over 75 or the latter for patients aged over 70. Radiotherapy offers useful palliation for superior mediastinal obstruction, chest pain, painful bony metastases and haemoptysis. Radical radiotherapy produces few long-term cures. Chemotherapy sometimes offers worthwhile life extension (a few months) in small-cell disease, which has usually metastasized at presentation. Early involvement of palliative care services (e.g. Macmillan cancer nurse in the UK) is important.

Malignant mesothelioma

This arises in the pleura and presents with chest pain, dyspnoea and bloody pleural effusion. The initial course may be indolent, high resolution CT scan may be helpful but diagnosis requires pleural biopsy. Because of the association with asbestos exposure and the long interval between exposure and presentation the effect of strict industrial regulation will not be apparent for years. Mesothelioma is increasing rapidly in prevalence, with an expected peak in 2015. It is important to diagnose; although management is palliative, compensation may be available — seek specialist advice.

Pulmonary fibrosis

The interstitial lung diseases are a group of disorders characterized by the abnormal accumulation of cells and/or non-cellular material within the walls of the alveoli. This results in thickening and stiffness of the elastic tissues of the lung, so that patients breathe in a rapid and shallow manner. The thickening of the alveolar walls decreases the efficiency of the transfer of oxygen. Many patients are short of breath on exertion and some have a troublesome dry cough. Fibrosis presents with breathlessness, widespread or bibasal fine crackles and sometimes clubbing. The course is generally progressive but the rate very variable, and some elderly patients will have had documented pulmonary fibrosis for a number of years.

Causes

- Idiopathic (cryptogenic fibrosing alveolitis, known as usual interstitial pneumonitis in the USA)
- Exposure—occupational, recreational or drugs (amiodarone, nitrofurantoin, gold)
- Secondary—connective-tissue diseases, sarcoidosis
- Focal—previous TB, radiotherapy

Carbon monoxide poisoning

Incidence
- Accounts for 40 000 emergency room attendances in the USA per year.
- Attributed to cause the death of 50 people per year in the UK.

Causes

- Smoke inhalation
- Faulty heating appliances
- Poor ventilation of such appliances
- Deliberate inhalation of car exhaust fumes; less common in older people

Clinical features and sequelae
- Carbon monoxide (CO) reduces oxygen delivery to tissues by two effects: it has an affinity for haemoglobin 220 times greater than that of

oxygen, and it shifts the oxyhaemoglobin dissociation curve to the left.
- CO also binds to intracellular proteins, causes activation of neutrophils leading to lipid peroxidation and may cause apoptosis in brain.
- Patients are hypoxic but not cyanosed. The skin and mucous membranes may appear 'cherry red'.
- Mild exposure (carboxyhaemoglobin (COHb) < 30%): headache, lethargy, nausea and vomiting.
- Moderate exposure COHb 50–60%: tachycardia, tachypnoea, syncope and fits.
- High exposure COHb > 60%: cardiorespiratory failure and death.
- CNS tissue damage can progress leading to neuropsychiatric problems up to 80 days post-exposure, including Parkinsonism, akinetic mutism, as well as acute confusion.

Management and prevention
- The key is to think about the possibility of CO poisoning and to take an arterial sample to check the level of carboxyhaemoglobin.
- Give 100% oxygen via a facemask.
- Do not be mislead by pulse oximeter readings: the pulse oximeter cannot distinguish between COHb and HbO_2.
- Consider hyperbaric oxygen early on in severe cases.
- Treat fits with intravenous diazepam.
- Prevention is obviously important. CO alarms are readily available. In the UK, landlords are legally required to have all domestic gas appliances checked annually by an approved engineer.

Further information

American Lung Association website—large number of lung conditions described in detail for patients and clear for students! http://www.lungusa.org/diseases/
British Lung Foundation website: http://www.lunguk.org/
Chief Medical Officer's Letter: *The Forgotten Killer:* www.doh.gov.uk/cmo/cmo98_5.htm
Omni—list of superb sites at Omni: http://omni.

ac.uk/browse/mesh/detail/C0024109L0024109.html#1

McGill Virtual stethoscope: If you are feeling a bit rusty about examining the respiratory system and interpreting what you hear try the McGill Virtual stethoscope! http://sprojects.mmip.mcgill.ca/MVS/MVSTETH.HTM

Walker, E. & Hay, A. (1999) Carbon monoxide poisoning. *British Medical Journal* **319**, 1082–3.

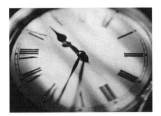

Gastrointestinal Disease and Nutrition

Introduction

Gastrointestinal (GI) symptoms are common throughout life—and the elderly are certainly not excluded. Structural changes, e.g. hiatus hernia, diverticular disease and gallstones, all increase with increasing age. Functional changes also increase, e.g. motility problems in the oesophagus and large bowel and falling acid secretion in the stomach. Almost one-fifth of patients presenting at a geriatric outpatient clinic will have GI problems.

Age changes

1 Impairment of sense of smell and taste.
2 Loss of teeth (see Chapter 15).
3 Impaired co-ordination of swallowing and oesophageal peristalsis.
4 Reduced gastric acid secretion.
5 Reduced pancreatic function due to duct and parenchymatous changes.
6 Increased development of diverticula.
7 Reduced surface area in small bowel.
8 Reduced large-bowel motility.

Weight loss

1 *Ageing changes*. There would appear to be a natural tendency to weight loss in old age

(in contrast to the weight gain so common in middle age)—due to a reduction in body-water content, bone loss (osteoporosis), thinning of connective tissue and the conversion of muscle to fat. However, those who maintain their lean body mass as they advance into old age have a better life expectancy than their shrinking peers.

2 *Systemic disease*. Weight loss is associated with all chronic disorders, e.g. chronic obstructive airway disease, cardiac failure, chronic renal failure, and with malignancy in all sites. Undiagnosed poorly controlled diabetes mellitus thyrotoxicosis and Addison's disease are other examples.

3 *Psychiatric disease*. The apathy of depression and the impaired insight and self-neglect in some demented patients will lead to attrition. The paranoia of a psychosis may make food unacceptable. The hyperactivity of some demented and hypomanic patients may result in weight loss. Alcohol abuse should also be considered.

4 *Iatrogenic disease*. Impaired appetite due to unpalatable treatment, e.g. spironolactone, or due to side-effects caused by toxicity or side effects, e.g. digoxin and levodopa, both potentially causing vomiting. Antidepressants and erythromycin cause nausea, and ACE inhibitors, loss of taste or an unpleasant taste. Diarrhoea due to misoprostol or antibiotic treatment.

5 *GI disease*:
(a) Dysphagia.
(b) Dyspepsia.
(c) Malabsorption.

Dysphagia

1 Problems in mouth (see Chapter 15).
2 Neuromuscular causes.
3 Pressure on the oesophagus.
4 Narrowing due to change in the wall.
5 Epithelial causes.
6 Intraluminal obstruction.

Neuromuscular dysphagia

1 Ageing (presbyoesophagus). Unco-ordinated oesophageal contractions or reduced activity.
2 Cerebrovascular disease including pseudo-bulbar palsy—see Chapter 7.
3 Bulbar palsy, e.g. motor-neuron disease.
4 Parkinson's disease. Akinesia complicates swallowing—may respond to levodopa and speech-therapy techniques. About 25% of patients are affected. Autonomic nervous system dysfunction also common.
5 Myasthenia gravis. Rare but important, because of good response to specific treatment with anticholinesterases.
6 Achalasia. More a problem of younger and middle-aged patients but may be an aspect of presbyoesophagus.
NB: nasogastric (NG) tube feeding is usually only justified on a short-term basis when recovery can be reasonably expected. Fine bore tubes should be used and only when the patient is aware of the problems and will, with help, be able to co-operate in this form of management—especially if long-term treatment is contemplated. See Chapter 7 for gastrostomy.

External pressure on the oesophagus

1 Pharyngeal pouches. All pouches become more common with increasing age. Zenker's diverticulum through the posterior pharyngeal wall at the upper level of the cricopharyngeus may result from inco-ordinated contractions. When large and full, it may hinder normal passage down the oesophagus. X-ray diagnosis is safest—endoscopy can be dangerous. Large and symptomatic pouches should be removed surgically and endoscopic techniques permit operations on frailer patients. More rarely, pouches may also occur at lower levels in the oesophagus.
2 Superior mediastinal obstruction. Secondary to malignancy (usually carcinoma of the bronchus) may be complicated by dysphagia.
3 Dilatation of the left atrium, especially in severe heart disease, can lead to dysphagia. A simple CXR, in conjunction with clinical signs, will usually be sufficient to make the diagnosis.
4 Aortic-arch dilatation.

Changes in the oesophageal wall
Barrett's oesophagus and carcinoma
Death rates from these conditions have risen dramatically in the past 30 years:
• Carcinoma of the oesophagus: 3–6/100 000.
• Carcinoma at junction: 1.5–3/100 000.
• Barrett's adenocarcinoma: 0.3–2.3/100 000.
Troublesome acid reflux is a risk factor common to all three conditions.

Barrett's oesophagitis has a high rate of conversion to malignancy, up to 150 times the normal rate. Ten per cent of cases have evidence of adenocarcinoma at the time of initial diagnosis. However, most patients die of other diseases. Regular surveillance is recommended in those patients who are otherwise fit: every 3 months for those with evidence of high-grade dysplasia, 6 months to 1 year for those with evidence of low-grade dysplasia and every 5 years for the remainder. Patients at particular risk of malignant change are those with a stricture, an ulcer or a segment greater than 80 mm.

Carcinoma of the oesophagus is the most important diagnosis (incidence on the increase and twice as common in men as in women). Position can usually be well localized by the patient's symptoms, which are likely to arise when two-thirds of the lumen is closed. Problems with solids, therefore, are the first and most important clue. X-ray is safest for diagnosis and great care is needed during endoscopy because of risk of perforation (results of X-ray examination should always be available prior to endoscopy). Endoscopy allows biopsy when the nature of the lesion is in doubt.

Treatment

Results are generally poor but palliation is valuable.

1 Surgery—for lesions at the lower end.
2 Radiation—for lesions at the upper end.
3 Stent insertion—when other measures are unjustified; complications with this method are common and obstruction is likely to occur at a later date.

Inflammatory lesions of the epithelium

1 *Oesophagitis*—with or without stricture, usually at the lower end and associated with hiatus hernia and acid reflux; therefore long previous history may be given. Endoscopy is the best diagnostic approach and allows biopsy to be taken (essential if any suspicion of malignant change), and also enables recognition of Barrett's oesophagus (gastric mucosa in the oesophagus).

Peptic oesophagitis may be treated with antacids. H2 antagonists may be needed in resistant cases. Proton-pump inhibitors (omeprazole) now treatment of choice. Strictures should be dilated.

2 *Oesophageal moniliasis*—the frail elderly are at risk, especially those who have received antibiotics, use steroid inhalers or are immunosuppressed. The typical white patches of thrush are often (but not always) present in the mouth. Endoscopy or barium swallow needed for confirmation of the oesophageal involvement. Fluconazole is the treatment of choice.

Intraluminal obstruction

Impacted objects may include food (especially if not properly chewed), missing dentures and other foreign bodies. Cognitively impaired patients are particularly at risk.

Dyspepsia

1 Indigestion is common at all ages (30% of the population) and 2–3% of prescribed drugs are antacids.
2 In many elderly patients the symptoms are very vague and non-specific and diagnosis, therefore, becomes increasingly difficult.
3 The lesions potentially responsible for indigestion become more common in old age.
4 Late-onset dyspepsia should be taken seriously and investigated by endoscopy.
5 *Helicobacter pylori* infection rises with age (up to 60% of elderly people are infected) and should be treated if demonstrated by either biopsy, culture, breath test or antibody test.

Lesions potentially responsible for indigestion

- Hiatus hernia: 60% over 70 years of age
- Peptic ulceration: 20% over 70 years of age
- Gallstones: 38% over 70 years of age
- Pancreatic disease
- Mesenteric ischaemia
- Carcinoma of large bowel
- Carcinoma of stomach
- Gastritis (especially drug-induced)

6 Many of these conditions are asymptomatic, e.g. 20% of hiatus hernia and up to 50% of gallstones.
7 Many patients will have more than one possible cause for their non-specific indigestion—a therapeutic trial may be the only way of identifying the responsible lesion.
8 Endoscopy is the investigation of first choice (except in the presence of dysphagia) and very acceptable for most elderly patients—care will be needed with pre-medication in those with poor respiratory reserve. Endoscopic retrograde cholangiopancreatography is most helpful in elderly patients with biliary-tract

disease and stones, if not too large, can be removed directly.

9 Ultrasound examination is the best technique for suspected gallbladder and pancreatic disease.

10 Special attention will be required when treatment is started, e.g.:

   (a) Metoclopramide—may precipitate or worsen extrapyramidal syndromes.

   (b) Cimetidine can cause mental confusion.

   (c) Aluminium salts should be avoided in constipated patients and magnesium in those with diarrhoea.

   (d) Bile salts have proved disappointing for dissolving gallstones—side-effects, especially diarrhoea, can be very troublesome in the elderly.

   (e) It has been suggested that long-term use of proton-pump inhibitors may lead to malignant change.

11 Many drugs cause dyspepsia; therefore drug history is a very important part of the investigation and assessment.

Gastrointestinal bleeding

Almost every recognized cause of GI bleeding becomes more common with increasing age:

  1 Hiatus hernia with oesophagitis.

  2 Gastritis—gastric erosions—elderly patients on NSAIDs have a sevenfold increased risk of bleeding compared with the same age group not taking such drugs.

  3 Duodenal ulcer and gastric ulcer.

  4 Carcinoma of the stomach (Fig. 11.1).

  5 Diverticular disease.

  6 Ischaemic bowel disease, sometimes difficult to differentiate from chronic inflammatory disease, e.g. Crohn's disease.

  7 Carcinoma of the large bowel.

  8 Piles.

  9 Colonic polyps—40% incidence in people aged over 65 years in a post-mortem study.

  10 Angiodysplasia of the colon.

Acute blood loss

Particularly dangerous in the elderly as the

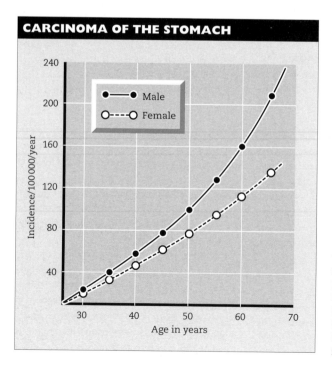

CARCINOMA OF THE STOMACH

Male
Female

Incidence/100 000/year

Age in years

Fig. 11.1 Carcinoma of the stomach. Special-risk groups are as follows: (i) old age (six times more common than in middle age); (ii) patients with pernicious anaemia (three to four times increased risk); (iii) previous gastric resection (five times as much risk); and (iv) patients with atrophic gastritis.

resulting hypotension may trigger problems in other systems, e.g. stroke, MI and renal failure. Speedy treatment is therefore required, initially blood transfusion but with quick and ready access to surgical intervention if the bleeding persists.

Acute upper GI bleeding in the elderly often presents as melaena without haematemesis — endoscopy may therefore be helpful in locating the site of bleeding and mucosal injection may help to stop bleeding.

Acute and severe ischaemia may present as rectal bleeding — but the ischaemia may be secondary to other pathology, e.g. a silent MI — a full assessment is therefore needed.

Chronic blood loss

Chronic GI bleeding is the most common cause of iron-deficiency anaemia in old age (see Chapter 14). The bleeding site will be asymptomatic in many patients. Investigation is therefore problematic — examination of both the upper and lower tract will be required in most cases and the ready acceptance of a simple benign lesion should not prevent further exploration for more serious causes — if the patient is sufficiently fit and co-operative to undergo extensive examination and subsequent treatment of any pathology.

Suggested plan of investigation
1 Confirmation of iron-deficiency anaemia.
2 Confirmation of GI bleeding — faecal occult bloods now less commonly performed.
3 Endoscopy of upper tract — to reveal or exclude oesophagitis and gastritis, as well as definite ulceration and malignancy. Barium swallow/meal is more appropriate if dysphagia is a problem.
4 Sigmoidoscopy followed by barium enema to study large bowel — preferably as an in-patient in frail elderly patients to ensure adequate bowel preparation. CT of the abdomen is kinder and almost as effective in frail elderly patients or those unable to co-operate with a barium enema.
5 Colonoscopy if barium enema or CT is

inconclusive — may confirm abnormality previously seen or reveal angiodysplasia.
6 Radioisotope-labelled red cells may be used to confirm presence and site of GI bleeding in difficult cases of brisk intermittent bleeding from unknown site.

Treatment
1 Specific treatment for underlying cause.
2 Oral iron supplements — ferrous sulphate if tolerated.
3 Transfuse only if haemoglobin is very low, e.g. less than 7 g, and patient unwell; take care if risk of congestive heart failure present.

The acute abdomen

A difficult diagnostic problem at all ages but even more so in old age. The mortality rate in elderly patients is much higher and may exceed 50% in some instances; there are four possible reasons for such depressing results:
1 Delay in presentation.
2 Atypical presentation ('silent').
3 Reluctance to operate on frail elderly patients.
4 Precipitation of other significant pathology during the acute episode, e.g. MI and stroke.
For pathology found in patients aged over 75 years undergoing emergency abdominal surgery, see Table 11.1.

Useful pointers in the elderly acute abdomen
1 Check hernial orifices.
2 X-ray for fluid levels, free air in peritoneal cavity, and distended bowel (e.g. sigmoid volvulus).
4 Check amylase level — about half the patients with acute pancreatitis are over 60 years of age.
5 Monitor presence of pulses and use ultrasound for detection of aortic aneurysm.
NB: Always consider the diagnosis of 'acute abdomen' in 'shocked', elderly patients, if supporting evidence is found on examination and emergency investigation; act quickly if surgical help is indicated.

ABDOMINAL PATHOLOGY

Diagnosis	No.	Mortality rate (%)
Strangulated hernia	115	16.5
Intestinal obstruction	103	37.9
Perforated peptic ulcer	22	40.9
Perforated large bowel	22	63.6
Ruptured aortic aneurysm	9	77.7
Biliary-tract disease*	22	
Mesenteric ischaemia*	10	

*Reduced numbers as some patients were treated conservatively.

Table 11.1 Acute abdomen — pathology in elderly patients undergoing surgery.

Bowel ischaemia

1 Twenty per cent of cardiac output is used to supply the GI tract—therefore any significant change in cardiac output is likely to affect the perfusion of the bowel and precipitate ischaemia.

2 At least two major mesenteric arteries must be compromised for bowel ischaemia to occur.

3 Because of a poor anastomotic arrangement, the left side of the colon is the most vulnerable segment of the bowel.

Clinical course

1 *Mild*:
  (a) Post-prandial abdominal pain, diarrhoea and weight loss.
  (b) Mucosal swelling—'thumb printing' on barium studies.
  (c) Recovery plus or minus scarring (stricture).

2 *Severe*:
  (a) Sudden severe pain—but may be 'silent'.
  (b) Movement of fluid into lumen, vomiting, diarrhoea and shock.
  (c) Ischaemic bowel wall allows bacteria to cross from lumen to peritoneum—peritonitis plus or minus septicaemia.
  (d) Death almost certain.

Treatment

• Acute/mild—support and treat underlying cause to prevent recurrence.

• Acute/severe—consult surgeons regarding resection; supportive and symptomatic treatment.

• Chronic—small frequent meals; correct any nutritional deficiencies due to malabsorption.

Diarrhoea

A very incapacitating condition in old age, especially if the patient is already disabled and immobile due to other pathologies.

1 *Spurious*, i.e. obstruction with overflow, must be excluded first by rectal examination, with or without sigmoidoscopy. The cause may be simple, e.g. faecal impaction, or serious, e.g. carcinoma of the rectum.

2 *Infective*—cultures must be taken and patient isolated while results awaited:
  (a) Viral—most common, usually self-limiting and supportive measures only required.
  (b) Bacterial—antibiotics only justified if patient's condition is grave; in mild cases they may prolong symptoms. May be endemic in hospital (e.g. *Clostridium difficile*).

3 *Inflammatory*—Crohn's disease of large bowel most common chronic inflammatory bowel disease in old age; diagnosis by biopsy and barium studies. Radioisotope white-cell scan also useful for determining extent of disease.

4 *Metabolic*—uncommon but exclude thyrotoxicosis; some cases secondary to diabetic neuropathy.

5 *Iatrogenic*—antibiotic diarrhoea common, especially after use of cephalosporins; purgative misuse; gastrectomy/vagotomy.

Constipation

Fear of becoming constipated is an aspect of old age that is more common than the genuine symptom. Seventy per cent of elderly people have their bowels open once daily, 11% every other day and 14% twice daily. Difficulty in passing motions is of greater importance than frequency of defaecation.

Causes of constipation are:

1 Faulty habits—low-residue diet, low fluid intake, lack of exercise and neglect of call to stool.
2 Poor appetite.
3 Immobility.
4 Drugs—analgesics, anticholinergics and diuretics.
5 Metabolic—myxoedema, hypercalcaemia.
6 Psychiatric—depression, dementia.
7 Functional—irritable bowel, purgative abuse (cathartic colon).
8 Pain—piles and fissures.

Management of constipation

1 Identify the nature and duration of constipation (small, hard stools are often related to low-fibre diet or dehydration; soft stools in a dilated rectum are suggestive of chronic laxative abuse).
2 Identify any precipitating causes, e.g. drugs, or bowel, endocrine or metabolic disease.
3 A rectal examination must be performed and recorded in the medical notes before prescribing laxatives.
4 If impaction is imminent—enemas are required.
5 If not impacted but a quick result is required—prescribe a stimulant (senna); occasionally an osmotic laxative (magnesium sulphate) will be required.
6 For short-term treatment (associated with acute illness)—ensure an adequate fluid intake and mobilize as soon as possible. Prescribe senna if stools bulky and soft; co-

danthrusate/co-danthramer if stools small and hard in association with opiates, otherwise liquid paraffin and magnesium hydroxide emulsion (milpar) may be an acceptable alternative.

7 Review the continuing need for laxatives once the patient is over the acute illness. Only prescribe laxatives on discharge from hospital if need continues, e.g. prior usage or continuing precipitant.
8 For longer-term treatment—high-fibre diet, attention to fluid intake and exercise may be all that is required.
9 For longer-term treatment where non-drug treatment fails or is impractical—prescribe a stool softener (co-danthrusate) or a bulking agent (ispaghula husk).
10 For intractable constipation—try a combination of treatments.
11 For patients on regular opiates—titrate co-danthrusate/co-danthramer against response.
12 The higher cost of lactulose can only be justified in those patients with chronic constipation in whom a bulking agent has failed.

Change in bowel habit

Alternating diarrhoea and constipation is always a worrying symptom. Carcinoma of the large bowel must be excluded but diverticular disease or large-bowel ischaemia and irritable colon are more common.

Barium-enema examination can be an ordeal in frail elderly patients. Best results are obtained if the patient is admitted for good bowel preparation and sigmoidoscopy before the procedure. Examination by CT is easier on the patient and performed as an out-patient procedure.

Faecal incontinence

1 Spurious diarrhoea due to faecal impaction (sometimes beyond rectal examination) is the commonest cause, especially in demented patients.
2 Circumstantial, i.e. intestinal hurry plus

physical immobility may lead to faecal incontinence. Treat underlying causes and reduce distance to toilet or commode.

3 Neurological or structural, e.g. paraplegia or rectal prolapse. Treat underlying cause where possible, e.g. surgery for rectal prolapse. If cure impossible — cause constipation with codeine phosphate and bulking preparations and relieve bowels at regular intervals with enemas.

4 Disinhibition and lack of insight, e.g. in dementia. Use bulking preparations and encourage regular toileting habits. In institutions facilitate recognition of toilet (e.g. large visible signs or brightly coloured lavatory door); protective clothing if all else fails.

Absorption

1 Small-bowel function declines with age but nutritional deficiencies only occur when additional factors intervene, e.g. poor diet or ill health.

2 Causes of malabsorption in youth may also occur *de novo* in old age, e.g. adult coeliac disease.

3 Maldigestion is more common than malabsorption, e.g. due to pancreatic disease.

4 Bacterial change in the small-bowel lumen due to stasis or diverticular disease is common (10% of elderly people) and is frequently clinically significant.

5 Ischaemia is a special cause of malabsorption in old age.

6 Iatrogenic causes must always be considered, e.g. post-gastrectomy, alcohol and some drugs, e.g. biguanides.

Possible indicators of malabsorption

1 Weight loss in spite of good dietary intake.
2 Low serum albumin level.
3 Unexplained iron-deficiency anaemia (with negative faecal occult blood).
4 Macrocytic anaemia.
5 Osteomalacia.
6 Obvious steatorrhoea is uncommon.

Potential causes of malabsorption in old age

The investigation of malabsorption in old age is very difficult and unsatisfactory but the following possibilities should always be considered and explored wherever possible:

1 Previous gastrectomy.
2 Small-bowel diverticular disease.
3 Altered luminal bacterial flora.
4 Pancreatic disease — causes maldigestion and steatorrhoea.
5 Adult coeliac disease.
6 Lymphoma.
7 Crohn's disease.
8 Mesenteric ischaemia.
9 Drugs, e.g. biguanides, cholestyramine.

Coeliac disease

This should no longer be considered as only a disease of childhood. Most cases present in the 5th decade and new cases have arisen as late as the 9th decade. In the UK, it now affects 1 in 200 of the population.

The development of antibody assays, endomysial and antigliadin, have made the detection of the condition much easier. The tests are done on blood samples and there is evidence of increasing frequency of positive results at least until the age of 60; beyond that age we have no further information. The endomysial antibody is the most specific but the diagnosis should still be confirmed wherever possible by a small bowel biopsy (biopsy negative cases do, however, exist).

The condition may be associated with other autoimmune conditions, i.e. thyroid, diabetes, primary biliary cirrhosis and Sjogren's syndrome. There is also evidence of association with neurological conditions including epilepsy, ataxia and dementia.

A period of treatment with a gluten free diet should be tried. The patient will be best placed to decide if the inconvenience of the diet outweighs any benefit gained in feelings of general well-being. Any deficiencies found at the time of diagnosis should be immediately corrected. The prophylactic aspect of dietary treatment (protection from malignant change) is of less importance in elderly patients than in the young.

For main presenting symptoms in elderly patients see Table 11.2.

Jaundice

• Surgical causes are common and must be identified rapidly before the condition becomes irremediable, ultrasound examination is the investigation of first choice.
• Medical causes of jaundice should be investigated and treated as in younger patients.
• Primary biliary cirrhosis and chronic hepatitis are more common in elderly patients than appreciated. Although occult, their prognosis in late life is often better than in younger patients.

Gastrointestinal malignancy

Oesophagus
See p. 96.

Gastric carcinoma
Although declining in incidence, it is still quite common; the rate for men is about twice that for women. The peak incidence is in the 8th decade (see Fig. 11.1) and most patients have advanced disease at diagnosis; it is therefore important to investigate late-onset dyspepsia. There is a genetic predisposition and an association with blood group A, atrophic gastritis and infection with H. pylori. Also there is considerable geographical variation in incidence and prognosis. It is particularly prevalent in Japan but the outlook for the disease there is more favourable; earlier diagnosis, which 'improves' survival time, may account for some of this but other factors are probably operating as well. Prolonged use of proton pump inhibitors may expose the patient to the risk of developing malignant change.

Clinically, indigestion, weight loss, vomiting, haematemesis, melaena and abdominal pain may occur. The diagnosis is confirmed by endoscopy or barium meal, and spread can be assessed by ultrasound or CT. The prognosis is poor and the treatment usually palliative; it may include gastrectomy, with adjuvant chemotherapy and radiotherapy or a bypass procedure.

Carcinoma of the pancreas
The incidence of pancreatic cancer is increasing in most developed countries although paradoxically not in Japan. It affects especially elderly men. Aetiological factors include cigarette smoking, high dietary fat and occupational exposure in the chemical and metal industries. The cancer is almost always far advanced at diagnosis and the prognosis is grim. Weight loss is usually striking and there may or may not be abdominal pain.

An ultrasound scan is a good initial investigation but CT is better able to define the extent of the growth. In most cases the head of the pancreas is involved, leading to obstructive jaundice. Radical surgery is usually not an option but

COELIAC DISEASE
Presenting symptoms in elderly patients
Diarrhoea or constipation
Apthous ulcers or sore mouth
Dyspepsia/abdominal discomfort
Fatigue
Bone pain
Weakness
Family history
Neuro/psychiatric syndromes

Table 11.2

stenting procedures provide relief from the symptoms of biliary obstruction.

Carcinoma of the colon and rectum

Colorectal cancer is the most common malignancy of the GI tract and the second most common cause of death from cancer in the UK; it is rare in Africa and Asia. This adenocarcinoma has a much lower grade of malignancy than gastric or pancreatic cancer, yet the 5-year survival of newly diagnosed cases is less than 30%. Patients with Crohn's disease and more especially those with polyposis and chronic ulcerative colitis are at increased risk of developing colorectal cancer (see also Table 11.3).

The clinical presentation is often rather vague, but malaise, abdominal pain and change of bowel habit, rectal bleeding, tenesmus or faecal incontinence, depending on the site of the lesion, are the usual pointers. Up to 29% present as obstruction — they have a poor prognosis — with less than 20% having a 5-year survival and 40% have secondaries at the time of presentation. The diagnosis is confirmed by rectal examination and sigmoidoscopy, followed by abdominal CT and/or colonoscopy or barium enema.

Treatment is surgical resection, ideally by a specialist colorectal surgeon. The use of self-expanding intraluminal stents looks promising, especially in obstructive cases of carcinoma of the colon.

The possibility of screening programmes, based on occult-blood detection and other techniques, is currently being pursued: see Table 11.4.

RISK FACTORS FOR CARCINOMA OF THE COLON

High red meat and animal fat intake.
Low fibre intake from fruit and vegetables.
Low physical activity.
Obesity
Genetic tendency

NB: Hormone replacement therapy may be protective.

Table 11.3

SCREENING FOR CARCINOMA OF THE COLON

Faecal occult blood	Test annually or bi-annually
	Detects about 70% of cases
	False positives lead to anxiety and unnecessary investigations
Flexible sigmoidoscopy	Well tolerated
	Detects about 80% of cases
Barium enema	Safe but requires good bowel preparation and may miss small lesions
Colonoscopy	In expert hands, detects almost 100% of cases
	Expensive
	Requires bowel preparation
	Has risk of complications

Table 11.4

Clinical nutrition

The importance of food in the maintenance and recovery of health is once again being recognized. The connection between nutrition and health was more obvious to past practitioners. The current obsession with high-tech medicine has deflected our attention away from such simple but important factors in health care.

General nutritional standards in elderly people in the UK

The majority of elderly people living in their own homes within the UK enjoy a reasonable diet. Their standards and practices are likely to be higher than younger members of our society. Elderly people (even old men) usually know how to cook and take a reasonably varied and balanced diet maintaining the good habits of their earlier lives.

The 1997/98 National Survey of Elderly People in the UK gave reassuring results. However, compared with the survey 30 years previously, the Medical Research Council found that people were eating less (energy intake was down 15%) but were increasing in weight. In 1997/98, 66% were considered overweight and only 5% underweight. The fat content of the diet was only slightly over the recommended levels but sugar was 7% above recommendations at 18%. All but up to 8% were taking sufficient vitamins and minerals; however, blood levels for folate, iron and vitamin C were subnormal in 10–15%.

Factors which impair dietary intake

- Illness — the most common and most serious
- Poor dental state — restricts dietary choice
- Poverty
- Being male
- Living in the North, especially Scotland
- Being in an institution

Percentage of elderly people regularly taking common foods

- Potatoes and bread: 70%
- Cooked vegetables: 66%
- Salads, raw vegetables and fruit: 50%
- Nutritional supplements: 30%

Subnutrition

In the UK subnutrition is rarely due to poverty; it is more likely to be a consequence of eccentricity, illness or loneliness. Overnutrition, with excess of carbohydrate, fat and calories, is of greater frequency than malnutrition and these excesses are often associated with a deficient amount of dietary fibre. Displacement of nutrients by alcohol abuse is another significant cause for dietary distortion. Other important factors related to diet in old age are as follows:

- The incidence of subnutrition is difficult to determine as dietary assessment by recall (of foods eaten) or weighed surveys are unreliable in many elderly subjects and particularly in the most vulnerable.
- There is considerable doubt about the accuracy of recommended intakes — elderly people may need more or less than some other groups.
- Surveys in the UK indicated levels of malnutrition of about 3–7%.
- Poor diets may be either the result or the cause of declining health.
- Other factors are social isolation and bereavement.
- Low blood levels of vitamins, etc. are common in old age, especially in the frail elderly, but their significance is uncertain (Table 11.5).
- Hyperhomocysteinaemia is associated with low folate and vitamin B_{12} levels and increased rates of vascular disease and thromboembolism.

Causes of nutritional deficiency

1 Inability to shop or to prepare food, e.g. in cases of dementia, depression, poverty, loneliness, eccentricity, blindness or immobility due to arthritis or neurological disease.

SUBNUTRITION

	Incidence
Haemoglobin <12 g	Up to 40% in institutions
	6–9% elderly at home
Serum iron	Approx. 20%
Red cell folate	Approx. 20%
Serum B_{12}	Approx. 20%
Red cell B_6	Approx. 6%
Vitamin C	Up to 50%
Vitamin D	Up to 70%

NB: Wide variation due to different groups studied and methods used—all incidences of low levels are more common than actual evidence of clinical deficiencies.

Table 11.5 Incidence of low blood levels of vitamins, etc. that have been reported in elderly subjects.

2 Impaired appetite which may be part of the clinical picture of general malaise, may be due to biochemical abnormalities, be a consequence of the side-effects of drugs or indicate underlying GI disease.

3 Malabsorption.

A simple recipe for a good diet

- Eat wholemeal bread not white bread.
- Have two portions of fresh vegetables daily.
- Eat three items of fresh fruit each day.
- Use $\frac{1}{2}$ L (1 pint) of semi-skimmed milk daily, for drinking and for use in cooking.
- Have one egg per day.
- Have one portion of meat or fish per day (preferably oily fish).
- Drink at least 2 L of fluid a day.

Assessment of nutritional status in old age

This is a very difficult task but the following criteria have been found to be of value in some instances (all have drawbacks).
- Dietary history.
- Weight change.
- Height change.
- Skinfold thickness.
- Muscle power.

- Blood levels of nutrients.
- Clinical evidence of nutritional disease.
- BMI under 15 (twice demispan may be substituted for height).
- The Mini-Nutritional Assessment (MNA) combines measurements and answers to questions (see Table 11.5).
- Taken in isolation most of these abnormalities have multiple causes. A diagnosis of malnutrition can only be made if several abnormalities are found—the cause of the malnutrition must then be explored and, if possible, corrected.

Dietary deficiencies in old age

1 The most obvious are calories, protein and fluid.

2 Vitamin B group—refractory heart failure, macrocytic anaemia due to folate deficiency, also peripheral neuropathy, dementia, vascular disease and thromboembolism.

3 Vitamin C—scurvy.

4 Vitamin D—osteomalacia.

5 Iron.

6 Fibre—diseases of 'Western civilization'.

Treatment of subnutrition in the community

1 Improve general health—treat underlying conditions.

2 Supplement intake—meals on wheels, lunch-

eon clubs, meal preparation by home help, give vitamin supplements and high-calorie liquid diets.

3 Education of patients and carers.

Treatment of subnutrition in hospital

Up to 50% of elderly people admitted to hospital are under nourished. Many deteriorate further during their stay due to inappropriate foods and catering arrangements. The consequences are serious and lead to prolonged hospital stays due to:

1 Poor healing and recovery.

2 Increased risk of complications, e.g. infection and depression.

Attention needs to be paid at all times to:

1 Suitable foods, e.g. familiar, easy to swallow, enjoyable and energy rich.

2 Small and frequent feeds — not large, widely spaced boluses.

3 Assistance with feeding when necessary, e.g. food placed within reach, modified utensils, cutting up of food and encouragement from staff.

4 Artificial feeding when appropriate — see Chapter 16.

NB: Please note, these measures should also apply to catering arrangements in care homes.

Further information

Borum M.L. (Ed.) *Clinics in Geriatric Medicine,* Vol. 15.3, *Gastroenterology.* W.B. Saunders, 1999.

Gelb A.M. (Ed.) *Clinical Gastroenterology in the Elderly.* Dekker, 1996.

Thomas, D. (Ed.) *Clinics in Geriatric Medicine,* Vol. 18.4, *Undernutrition in Older Adults.* W.B. Saunders, 2002.

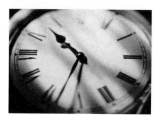

Disorders of Homeostasis and Metabolism

Age changes

There is a reduction in lean body mass and body water and usually a relative increase in fat (Fig. 12.1).

Endocrine changes

Some elderly people have unmeasurably low levels of growth hormone; in some, it fails to respond to an insulin tolerance test. Some male subjects have global muscle wasting, and the administration of human growth hormone has been shown to increase lean body mass and reduce adipose tissue but without clear benefit to quality of life.

Other hormonal changes include:
- Serum noradrenaline ↑ (but β-receptors ↓).
- Insulin ↑ (due to insulin resistance): carbohydrate tolerance diminishes.
- AVP ↓ susceptibility to hyponatraemia ↑.
- Atrial natriuretic peptide ↑ and nocturia ↑.
- Oestrogen and progesterone in women ↓, FSH and LH ↑.
- Testosterone in men ↓, FSH and LH ↑.
- Renin and aldosterone ↓.

Adenomas are common in anterior pituitary, thyroid and adrenal glands.

Fluid and electrolyte imbalance

Acutely unwell elderly patients are very often fluid-depleted or fluid-overloaded and, occasionally, both.

Reasons for vulnerability to dehydration:
1 Reduction in body water.
2 Inadequate intake due to:
  (a) Impaired thirst response.
  (b) Dementia or depression.
  (c) Immobility.
  (d) Reluctance through fear of being 'caught short'.
  (e) Swallowing difficulty.
  (f) Acute illness.
  (Mainly affects intracellular compartment, with thirst, confusion, drowsiness.)
3 Loss:
  (a) Reduced concentrating ability by kidney.
  (b) Diuretics.
  (c) Diabetes, diarrhoea and vomiting.
  (Loss of salt and water often replaced by water/tea, etc. Mixed salt and water depletion presents with confusion, weakness, loss of tissue, turgor, tachycardia, postural hypotension, as extracellular compartment mainly affected.)

Hyponatraemia

This is common in geriatric patients and is due to too little sodium, too much water or both. Do not treat the sodium level in isolation. Decide whether the patient is dehydrated, euvolaemic, or fluid overloaded.

If the patient is dry, salt and water has been lost either through the kidneys (diuretics especially thiazides, renal failure, osmotic diuresis), the gut (vomiting, diarrhoea, fistula, adenoma) or skin (burns).

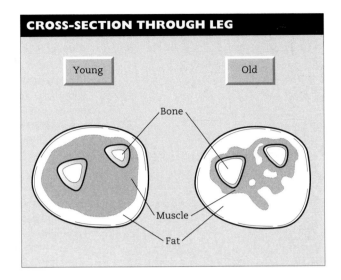

CROSS-SECTION THROUGH LEG

Young

Old

Bone

Muscle

Fat

Fig. 12.1 Diagramatic cross-section through a young and an old leg to show change in composition.

If the patient is oedematous there is relative water excess due to fluid retention (in cardiac failure, liver failure or nephrotic syndrome) or excess water intake (usually over-enthusiastic dextrose after surgery).

If the patient does not appear dry or wet, one of the above may be developing. However, if the urine is concentrated (sodium >20 mmol/L in the presence of hyponatraemia) and the plasma is dilute with a low plasma osmolality (<260 mmol/kg) the syndrome of inappropriate antidiuretic hormone (SIADH) is present. This leads to intracellular water accumulation in the brain with confusion, headache, lethargy, coma and fits.

Causes of SIADH

- Drugs, especially SSRIs, venlafaxine, opiates, certain sulphonylureas
- Malignancy
- CNS, e.g. stroke
- Chest disease, e.g. pneumonia

Treatment

- Underlying cause
- Water restriction/intravenous infusion of Normal saline as appropriate
- Demeclocycline (blocks action of ADH on tubule)

Hypernatraemia

This is usually due to water loss in excess of sodium loss and occurs where patients are unable to take in enough water to meet their needs.

Oedema

Not all oedema is heart failure and a knee-jerk prescription of diuretics may merely convert 'fluid in the ankles to urine in the slippers'. If oedema is present to the knee, in a patient in a chair slip a hand under the thigh and, if oedema is present there too, lean the patient forward to check for a sacral pad.

Some causes of ankle oedema

Raised venous pressure
- Gravity (prolonged sitting)
- Cardiac failure
- pelvic mass

The following causes are often unilateral
- Venous insufficiency (side of hip surgery)
- DVT
- Lack of muscle pump (side of hemiparesis)
- Over-active muscle pump in one leg (tremor in Parkinson's disease) makes bilateral oedema appear unilateral

Fluid retention
- Cardiac failure
- Drugs (NSAIDs, steroids, calcium channel blockers, glitazones)
- Renal failure

Hypoalbuminaemia
- Nutritional, hepatic disease or protein loss via kidney, bowels or extensive skin loss (dip stick urine for protein).

Lymphatic obstruction
- Usually malignant.
- Inflammatory.
- Localized.

Hypokalaemia

Another common finding in geriatric practice, often due to diuretic therapy or GI loss (remember the laxative abuser) but often at least partially due to inadequate dietary intake (many patients have diets deficient in fruit, vegetables and meat). It has been reported that sick elderly females, in particular, may be found to have 'acute transient hypokalaemia', which may be due to a shift into the cells and which usually self-corrects within a few days. Hypokalaemia exacerbates digoxin toxicity. Replace orally or by slow intravenous infusion if severe. If the response is poor, check for low magnesium, as correcting this helps.

Hyperkalaemia

This occurs in renal failure and rhabdomyolysis (both of which may follow a collapse and long lie). However, drugs are the common culprits. In old age, cardiac failure can often be managed with frusemide rather than the potassium retaining combination of frusemide and amiloride that is often needed in middle age. A combination of an ACE inhibitor and spironolactone may be evidence-based treatment for cardiac failure in drug trials but, particularly if Frumil® is also prescribed, will usually result in dangerous hyperkalaemia with older kidneys! Give intravenous calcium, insulin and glucose and calcium resonium.

Diabetes mellitus

Definition

The WHO (1999) (see NICE guidelines) advises that the range of blood glucose indicative of diabetes mellitus are as follows:
- Random venous plasma glucose $\geq$ 11.1 mmol/L *or*
- Fasting plasma glucose $\geq$ 7.0 mmol/L *or*
- Plasma glucose $\geq$ 11.1 mmol/L at 2 h after a 75-g oral glucose load (oral glucose tolerance test).

Epidemiology

Prevalence rises with age up to the highest age band studied (84 years) and is higher in Afro-Caribbean and Asian people than white people in the UK. It is estimated that 1.4 million people in the UK have diabetes, 80% of whom have Type 2 diabetes. Because of the ageing population and increase in obesity, this is predicted to rise to 3 million by 2010. Half the diabetic population and a quarter of insulin users are elderly. A common 'ballpark' figure is that 5% of people aged 70 have known diabetes and the same number have unrecognized impaired glucose tolerance.

Mechanism

The impairment of glucose intolerance in old age is mainly caused by reduced tissue sensitivity to insulin at post-receptor level. There is also beta cell dysfunction; the pancreas is also less able to secrete insulin in response to a glucose load and the rapid post-prandial spike of secretion is lost. The older diabetic usually has Type 2 diabetes, although the number of Type 1 graduates to old age will increase steadily. Occasionally, Type 1 diabetes occurs *de novo* in an older person.

Effects

Aged 65–75 diabetics have twice the cardiovascular and all-cause mortality — but thereafter it tends to revert towards normal. One-third have visual impairment, more often due to cataract than to retinopathy, the amputation rate is enormously increased and cognitive and psychosocial function is generally impaired. A common end-stage comprises poor cardiac function, renal failure and marked oedema.

Management

Management of the diabetes must be part of a holistic approach to cardiovascular risk and will depend greatly on the circumstances of the patient; a frail nursing home resident requires different care to an otherwise fit and independent 75 year old who should not be excluded from diabetic clinics.

Aims include a feeling of well-being and the avoidance of hypoglycaemia, which can cause brain damage or injury, but tight enough control to avoid complications in younger elderly patients. Haemoglobin A1C (HbA$_{1c}$) should be measured at 2–6 monthly intervals. Dietary advice concentrates on weight reduction in the obese, reducing fat intake and ensuring that carbohydrates are of a high-fibre, unrefined, polysaccharide type. Regular exercise is highly beneficial. Smoking must be discouraged, statins prescribed for hypercholesterolaemia (at least up to 80 years) and hypertension treated vigorously if the patient can tolerate this. ACE inhibitors may have a particular role to play if there is microscopic albuminuria. Patients require basic education about diabetes and how lifestyle changes will help if they are to adhere to their diet. Periodic surveillance, including eyes and feet, is at least as important as in younger subjects.

If drugs are necessary, following the United Kingdom Prospective Diabetes Study (UKPDS) metformin, which decreases gluconeogenesis and increases peripheral utilization of glucose, has become increasingly popular, whereas it used to be restricted to obese patients. Care must be taken if there is renal impairment (contraindicated if creatinine > 130 μmol/L) or risk of sudden renal deterioration. Sulphonylureas, which augment insulin secretion, are another option: those with short half-lives (e.g. glipizide 3–6 h) are favoured (avoid chlorpropramide and glibenclamide). Weight gain may be a problem. Glimepramide is a sulphonylurea marketed as a post-prandial glucose regulator. The α-glucosidase inhibitor acarbose, which delays starch absorption, is often not well tolerated because of flatulence. New drugs include repaglinide, a metiglinide and nateglinide, the first of a new group of glucose-responsive amino acid derivatives, which are both short-acting and restore early phase insulin secretion and reduce post-prandial glucose spikes. They may be useful in the elderly as there is little risk of hypoglycaemia. The new thiazolidinedione derivatives ('glitazones') work by activating the peroxisome proliferator activated receptor gamma (PPARγ) resulting in increased glucose uptake and utilization in the periphery. However, these are not recommended if there is co-existing heart failure, a common problem in the elderly diabetic, so experience is limited. Whatever drug is chosen, further education is essential to make sure the patient understands how and when to take the drug, and how to manage hypoglycaemia.

If control is poor, it is a mistake to be too reluctant to institute insulin, which makes the poorly controlled diabetic feel vastly better. However, the common twice-daily injection regime (of, for instance, Mixtard®) can pose practical difficulties in those living alone whose intellect, vision or dexterity is too limited to permit self-injection. Sometimes a single morning injection of Ultratard® achieves adequate control. Combinations of insulin and tablets are beginning to appear in clinical practice. Foot care and regular chiropody are particularly important in the elderly diabetic.

Hyperosmolar crisis

Other than this, diabetic crises and complications do not present any special features in old people. Hyperosmolar coma typically occurs in patients with Type 2 diabetes that has often hitherto caused very little problem. An osmotic diuresis leads to insidiously progressive dehydration and hypotension, culminating in stupor or coma. However, because there is still some endogenous insulin, the body does not switch to metabolic pathways resulting in ketone production. Extreme hyperglycaemia, hypernatraemia and uraemia are typical. The aim here is steady correction of the metabolic derangement. Avoid doing things too rapidly and remember rehydration is more important than insulin. It is safest to give Normal saline, as this will be relatively dilute in comparison with the plasma. Depending on the severity and the patient's cardiac status, give a litre over 1–2 h and assess the effect. Continue with a litre over 2 h, 4 h, 6 h, etc. It may be necessary to give 10 L of fluid over and above output over the first 48 h or so, ideally monitored by the central venous pressure (CVP) line. Wait an hour before giving any insulin, the glucose often falls dramatically with rehydration, but if it is needed 1 unit per hour would be a typical dose. The risk of venous thrombosis is high so give a full preventative dose of heparin (e.g. 40 mg Clexane®). Those who survive do not need insulin unless control remains poor.

Thyroid disease — function tests

Normal function is usually preserved until at least 80 years of age but in centenarians TSH and free T_3 levels may decline. In the seriously ill patient, the TSH, T_3 and T_4 levels may all be misleadingly low ('sick euthyroid syndrome'), and amiodarone and anticonvulsants often interfere with thyroid-function tests (TFTs). Always check TFTs before starting amiodarone and remember that this will interfere with ra-

dioiodine treatment. Both hypo- and hyperthyroidism are difficult to diagnose clinically in old age and many geriatricians routinely check TSH in any significant illness.

Hyperthyroidism

Presentation is atypical — AF, heart failure, weight loss, proximal myopathy, functional decline; thyroid nodular or impalpable — sometimes retrosternal. Treatment is carbimazole and a beta-blocker if the heart rate is high, prior to definitive therapy with I^{131}. Carbimazole can be given in a dose aiming for normal thyroid hormone level or in a dose to block all production with thyroxine replacement (see BNF 6.6.2). Remember to give written advice about sore throat on carbimazole (neutropaenia).

Hypothyroidism

Hypothyroidism affects 5% of people aged over 60 and it may be due to Hashimoto's disease, I^{131} treatment, surgery, or it may be idiopathic or, occasionally, secondary to pituitary failure. Clinical pointers include impaired cognition and slow-relaxing ankle jerks. Treatment is with thyroxine 25 μg, with similar increments every 3–4 weeks until on a daily dose of around 100 μg, the patient feels well and the TSH confirms euthyroidism.

Adrenal disease

Cushing's syndrome

The commonest cause in old age is iatrogenic. Older people are often left on higher doses of steroid than they need, particularly for polymyalgia rheumatica, which usually burns itself out after a couple of years. Older people on steroids are particularly prone to fluid retention, heart failure, diabetes, proximal myopathy and osteoporosis (always give bone protection), and high doses may lead to acute confusion, 'steroid psychosis'.

Addison's disease

Adrenal insufficiency may occur acutely, usually when there is an acute severe illness in a patient with iatrogenic adrenal suppression due to long-term steroid treatment. Chronic adrenal insufficiency is due to adrenal destruction, e.g. TB or metastases and not surprisingly (since the presentation is insidious even in middle age) has to be thought about in order to carry out a short Synacthen test.

Autonomic nervous system

The autonomic nervous system (ANS) is the part of the nervous system most closely involved in homoeostatic mechanisms, and it can become defective as a result of diabetes, Parkinson's disease, peripheral neuropathy, and, so they say, cerebrovascular disease, alcoholism, syphilis, thiamine deficiency and a variety of uncommon disorders. But probably, too, it can become defective in old age without any other identifiable neurological disorder. It is concerned in two particular homeostatic functions which have to do with physics rather than chemistry — control of body temperature and BP.

Accidental hypothermia

One day, the neighbours notice that an old lady who lives by herself has not taken the milk in or drawn back the curtains and there is no sign of life from her house. They have a key, so they let themselves in and, after shouting for her with no response, they eventually find her in her bedroom, on the floor, in a dazed condition, wearing only her nightie. Hesitant to move her, they call the GP and together they manage to get her into bed.

The GP notices that the room is cold—there is no heating and there is a window open. The GP checks that there is no obvious injury from the fall, such as a fractured neck of femur, that there is no obvious illness which may have caused her to fall, such as a hemiplegia, and assumes she may have had some debilitating illness, e.g. pneumonia, that made her collapse on the floor as she tried to get out of bed to visit the toilet. She is drowsy, croaky of voice, very slow of movement and response,

and her limbs are strikingly rigid. The GP puts a hand on her abdomen under her nightie and finds that it feels unnaturally cool. Her pulse rate is 50 b.p.m., her BP 100/70 and the tympanic thermometer reveals a core temperature of 31°C. **Why?**

1 It has been a cold March night.
2 She has a serious illness—pneumonia (drugs such as alcohol and phenothiazines also predispose to hypothermia).
3 She is only wearing a nightie and has spent most of the night on the floor.
4 Her ability to detect a falling ambient temperature is less good than that of a young person. The previous evening, she forgot to put on the woolly nightcap her thoughtful neighbour gave her for Christmas, not realizing that 40% of the body's heat is lost through the scalp. She also failed to close the window and to plug in the electric fan heater that her daughter had bought her. She has never had central heating installed.
5 As her body temperature started to fall, her ANS failed to cut down heat loss by cutaneous vasoconstriction and failed to increase heat production by shivering.

The three main factors which have combined to produce this typical clinical picture are: systemic illness, exposure to cold and ANS dysfunction; if sufficiently severe, only one of these factors need be present to cause accidental hypothermia (core temperature less than 35°C).

Clinical features
Above 32°C the features may be those of an underlying disease or of functional decline. Below 32°C the features are as described for the above patient and, below 27°C, 75% of patients are comatose. Pancreatitis, hypoglycaemia and ventricular arrhythmias are among the complications, and everyone seems to remember the J waves but you diagnose hypothermia with a thermometer, not an ECG. Over 30°C the mortality is about 33% but below 30°C it approaches 70%.

Management
At a core temperature just below 35°C, it is reasonable to re-warm the patient at home

and counsel (scold) to prevent recurrence. More serious cases (30–34°C) have traditionally received gradual passive re-warming in hospital at 0.5–1.0°C per hour to avoid sudden profound hypotension. Avoid instrumentation, which may precipitate serious arrhythmia. Below 30°C some would argue that conservative measures constitute losing tactics and that admission to the ITU is required for active re-warming, using a 'Bair hugger'. However, most elderly patients have to take their chance on an open ward.

Other dangers of extreme weather

Cold kills in other ways and in an average winter there are 40 000 deaths in England and Wales above the expected number, mainly due to vascular causes. Platelets, haematocrit, blood viscosity, plasma cholesterol and, in old men at least, systolic BP tends to rise on exposure to the cold. Blood fibrinogen levels may rise during the winter months. Slipping on icy pavements is a further hazard. The incidence of strokes and the mortality rate also tend to rise among elderly people in the UK during heat waves. Food poisoning is another hazard of heat waves.

Further information

Diabetes UK (formerly the British Diabetic Association) website has lots of information for patients, carers and professionals: http://www.diabetes.org. uk/ (use the search facility to check diagnostic criteria, the latest on the NSF, etc.)

Electronic British Medical Journal's collected resources website: http//bmj.com/cgi/collection/diabetes

Fall, P.J. (2000) Hyponatremia and hypernatremia. A systematic approach to causes and their correction. *Postgraduate Medicine* 107(5), 75–82.

NICE guidelines for the management of diabetes September 2002: http://www.nice.org.uk/ (search for diabetes)

Scottish intercollegiate guidelines website—this is a super website with a wide range of material. The diabetes guidelines do not specifically cover the elderly but feet are well dealt with! http://www.sign.ac.uk

United Kingdom Department of Health website with press releases explaining latest policies. Relevant examples here include 'Keep warm, keep well': http://www.doh.gov.uk

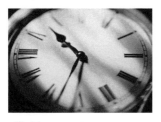

Genitourinary Disease

Ageing changes

1 In old age, renal function is reduced to about 50% of peak function (i.e. that at age of 30 years).
2 Serum urea in healthy old age remains normal in spite of falling renal function.
3 The aged kidney has impaired ability both to concentrate urine and to process an extra water load quickly. This is one explanation for the increased incidence of nocturia in old age. The ability to concentrate urine falls from 1300 to 850 mosm/L.
4 Renal scarring is evident in 46% of 'normal' elderly kidneys.
5 Reduced renal function is due to:
   (a) Nephron 'drop-out'. ⎫ Both exaggerated in
   　　　　　　　　　　　　 ⎬ hypertension, dia-
   (b) Vascular changes. ⎭ betes or pyeloneph-
   　　　　　　　　　　　　　ritis in earlier life
   (c) Poor response to ADH.
6 The combination of renal ageing changes and systemic or renal disease may lead to rapid and dramatic renal failure in elderly patients.
7 Atrophic changes occur in the urogenital tract of post-menopausal women.
8 Prostatic size increases with age.
9 The unstable bladder, with detrusor instability owing to sudden uncontrollable rise in bladder pressure due to contractions while filling, becomes increasingly common in old age, due to neurological degeneration.

Renal failure in old age

Pre-renal and post-renal causes are most frequently responsible for this presentation. Therefore management includes:
• Rehydrating the patient.
• Excluding renal-tract obstruction by examination and ultrasound.
• Excluding urinary tract infection by midstream urine.
• Intrinsic renal disease is not often of paramount clinical importance in geriatric patients but all medications should be scrutinized to omit those which damage renal function further and to reduce the doses of those excreted by the kidney.
• Age alone should not be used as a contraindication for renal dialysis. In fact, many elderly patients adopt a very philosophical approach, which makes them very suitable — especially for continuous ambulatory peritoneal dialysis (CAPD). Up to 20% of dialysis patients are aged over 70 years.

Intrinsic renal disease

1 Nephrotic syndrome. In a recent series of patients aged over 50 years with nephrotic syndrome (diabetics were excluded) the underlying cause in order of incidence was:
   (a) Membranous glomerulonephritis.
   (b) Proliferative glomerulonephritis.

(c) Amyloid: usually secondary to long-standing inflammatory disease, e.g. bronchiectasis, osteomyelitis or rheumatoid arthritis.

(d) Minimal-change glomerulonephritis.

2 Diabetic nephropathy. No special features in old age.

3 Myeloma: see Chapter 14.

4 Nephrocalcinosis/stones. Exclude vitamin D intoxication, gout and hyperparathyroidism — all occur more frequently in old age.

Infection

• Urinary-tract infections (bacteriuria greater than 10^5/mL) are common in old age.

• Twenty per cent of people over the age of 65 will experience a urinary tract infection.

• This increases to 50% of women in institutional care.

• Female to male ratio: 3 : 1.

• *Escherichia coli* is the most common pathogen. Others include *Proteus*, and *Klebsiella*.

• Asymptomatic bacteriuria with no pyuria does not require treatment.

• Pyelonephritis is responsible for 20% of cases of renal failure.

Precipitating factors for urinary tract infections in old age

1 High incidence of urinary stasis:
   (a) Poor bladder emptying.
   (b) Prostatism.
   (c) Bladder diverticula.

2 Hormonal changes affecting the mucous membranes of women.

3 Associated disorders:
   (a) Diabetes.
   (b) Atherosclerosis.
   (c) Immobility.
   (d) Indwelling catheter.

4 Urinary tract stones.

Unusual presentations of urinary-tract infection in old age

1 Asymptomatic, i.e. found on screening — should remain untreated if patient is well.

2 Acute confusional state — catheterization

may be required to obtain specimen; alternatively organism may on some occasions be obtained on blood culture.

3 New urinary incontinence.

4 Increasing drowsiness due to worsening renal failure.

Management

1 Culture organism from urine or blood.

2 Maintain good fluid input (greater than 2 L/day).

3 Give appropriate antibiotics (trimethoprim best 'blind treatment').

4 Reverse precipitating cause, if possible (see above).

Obstructive nephropathy

Obstructive nephropathy is secondary to a blockage anywhere along the urinary tract.

Lesion in urethra

1 Males (usually).

2 Past history of previous episodes of sexually transmitted disease.

3 Bladder palpable or demonstrable on ultrasound.

4 Catheterization is difficult or impossible, consider suprapubic approach, and obtain expert help.

Bladder-neck obstruction

Prostate pathology

1 By the 8th decade, 50% of prostates contain areas of benign nodular hyperplasia, chronic prostatitis, pre-malignant changes. The patient may complain of hesitancy, urgency, nocturia and poor stream.

2 Fewer than half of all men with benign prostatic hypertrophy develop symptoms. In mild cases or in patients who are a poor surgical risk, treatment with α-adrenoceptor antagonists (e.g. indoramin and doxazosin) may be beneficial. Newer, more selective alpha-blockers such as tamsulosin are said to be less likely to cause orthostatic hypotension.

3 Rectal examination first essential step in

diagnosis—enlargement may be confirmed by rectal ultrasound.

4 Only 1% of prostatic cancers cause problems during life but clinically are the second most frequent malignancy in men.

5 Any suspicious nodules should be biopsied to exclude carcinoma; this can be done transrectally.

6 Raised prostate specific antigen (PSA) supports the diagnosis of carcinoma; if this is very high, it suggests metastatic disease.

7 Transurethral prostatectomy (TURP) is the treatment of choice for benign prostatic hypertrophy (BPH) but there is increasing anxiety about safety (blood loss and absorption of irrigation fluids) and need for repeat surgery.

8 Treatment of carcinoma (orchidectomy, hormone therapy, radical surgery or radiotherapy) depends on the spread of the disease and patient's preferences.

9 In the case of the chance finding of malignant cells in a TURP specimen, the management remains problematic, many patients will live trouble-free.

Gynaecological problems—detectable on pelvic examination

1 Malignancy of female genital tract and presence of fibroids.

2 Hormone-deficient changes in mucosa of trigone of bladder.

Spread of rectal malignancy

Detectable on rectal examination and on CT scanning.

Faecal impaction

Must always be excluded, as it is readily reversible.

Neurological disease

Affecting bladder emptying.

Iatrogenic disease

Anticholinergic drugs such as tolterodine and oxybutinin are common precipitants.

Retroperitoneal disease

Malignancy and fibrosis (latter may be drug-induced, e.g. by beta-blockers and methysergide). It is usually associated with a very high ESR.

Unilateral disease

Due to ureteric obstruction, secondary to stones, malignancy or fibrosis.

Drugs and the kidneys

1 Nephrotoxic drugs:
  (a) Antibiotics, e.g. streptomycin, gentamicin and tetracycline.
  (b) Analgesics, e.g. NSAIDs, phenacetin.
  (c) Anti-rheumatics, e.g. penicillamine, gold.

2 Overdosage of drugs acting on kidneys, i.e. diuretics leading to dehydration, hypotension and electrolyte imbalance, to the extent of causing marked renal failure.

3 Renal changes causing drug toxicity, i.e. drugs excreted via the kidneys—best example is digoxin.

4 ACE inhibitors may precipitate renal failure if used in patients with silent renovascular disease.

Blood pressure and the kidneys

1 Renal disease may cause hypertension, e.g. chronic pyelonephritis.

2 The overtreatment of high blood pressure will impair renal function. Yet untreated hypertension may result in renal failure!

3 About one-third of elderly patients with hypertension have impaired renal function.

4 Hypotension, e.g. after bleeding, myocardial infarction or pulmonary embolus, may result in renal shutdown and acute renal failure especially where renal function is already compromised by extreme old age or pathological changes.

5 Renal artery stenosis (RAS) may first present as a marked deterioration in renal function after treatment with an ACE inhibitor.

6 Bilateral renal artery stenosis can also present as 'flash' pulmonary oedema which is thought be due to the combination of the RAS and fluid overload plus diastolic ventricular dysfunction.

Haematuria

See Table 13.1.

Urinary incontinence

Urinary incontinence is defined as 'the involuntary loss of urine sufficient in volume or frequency to be a social or a health problem'.
• It affects 50% of older people in hospital and nursing homes and 35% of those living in the community.

• It is often concealed by the patient because of embarrassment.
• Only 20% of affected women consult a doctor.
• It is twice as common in women as in men.
• This is because of the female anatomy, and because low oestrogen levels lead to reduced cohesiveness of the urethra making it patulous.

Complications
• Embarrassment leads to fear of going out and this leads to social isolation.
• Depression.
• Sexual problems.
• Huge burden on patients and their carers: financial (pads are expensive) and workload (extra washing).
• Increased risk of institutionalization.

CAUSES, INVESTIGATIONS AND MANAGEMENT OF HAEMATURIA

Cause	Investigations	Management
Bleeding diathesis	Abnormal clotting, low platelets	Review need for anticoagulants, check liver function
Urinary tract infection	MSU, blood cultures	Antibiotics, treat predisposing factors
Transitional cell carcinoma of the bladder	Cystoscopy	Transurethral resection of bladder tumour with regular review
Ureteric stones	IVU, ultrasound	Extracorporeal shockwave lithotripsy, endoscopic removal, preventative measures
Benign prostatic hypertrophy	Clinical examination	Alpha-blockers, TURP
Carcinoma of the prostate	Biopsy, PSA	Treat as appropriate
Intrinsic renal disease	Consider renal biopsy if appropriate	Treat as appropriate
Renal cell carcinoma	Ultrasound or CT abdomen, urine cytology	Treat as appropriate
Contamination with vaginal blood	Obtain clean catch specimen, with catheter if necessary	See Vaginal bleeding, p.120
Immune complex disease, e.g. bacterial endocarditis	Blood cultures, echocardiography, etc.	Treat underlying condition

Table 13.1

- Skin irritation and maceration may lead to pressure sores.

Reversible causes
The mnemonic '**diappers**' is helpful! See Table 13.2.

Types of incontinence
1 **Stress incontinence**: involuntary leaking of urine when sneezing, coughing, and exercising. Most common in multiparous women and those who have had pelvic surgery. In men the most common cause is sphincter damage after radical prostatectomy.

Non-surgical treatments: pelvic floor exercises (e.g. Kegel's exercise involves concentrating on contracting the pelvic floor to interrupt the flow of urine), ring pessaries

Surgical procedures: periurthral collagen injections, colposuspension, anterior repair for prolapse.

2 **Urge incontinence**: is frequent and urgent passing of small amounts of urine, sometimes with so little warning that the patient does not reach the toilet in time. This is due to detrusor instability. It increases with age and is associated with hyperreflexia in neurological conditions such as stroke, multiple sclerosis and Parkinson's disease.

Treatment: antimuscarinic anticholinergic agents such as oxybutinin and tolterodine. Tolterodine is said to be more specific and therefore cause less dry mouth and confusion.

3 **Overflow incontinence**: is most common in men with benign prostatic hypertrophy, but may also be secondary to prostatic carcinoma or urethral stricture. It is also associated with neurological deficits, e.g. diabetes.

If the cause is benign prostatic hypertrophy, *treatments* include alpha-blockers such as doxazosin and tamsulosin, or TURP.

An approach to incontinence
1 Start by asking the patient to keep a voiding diary, recording whether they are continent or incontinent throughout the day, plus other symptoms to help diagnose the type of incontinence.

2 Examine the abdomen for a palpable bladder secondary to obstruction.

3 Rectal examinations to assess prostate size in men, exclude faecal impaction and check integrity of anal sphincter.

4 In women, vaginal examination to exclude senile vaginitis and prolapse.

5 Neurological examination to exclude cord problems.

REVERSIBLE CAUSES OF URINARY INCONTINENCE

	Investigations	Management
Delirium	MSU, CXR, FBC, U & Es	Treat underlying cause
Infection	MSU	Treat infection
Atrophic urethritis		Topical oestrogen in females
Pharmaceuticals: Sedatives, caffeine diuretics antidepressants, alcohol		Use alternatives if possible, try lower doses
Psychiatric: secondary to dementia, behavioural problems		Exclude treatable causes, toilet regularly
Excess urine production	Serum glucose, calcium	Treat diabetes, hypercalcaemia
Restricted mobility	Joint and neurological examination	Physiotherapy, walking aids, commode, disabled toilets
Stool impaction	Rectal examination	Regular laxatives, adequate fluid intake

Table 13.2

6 Assess medications; are there alternatives?

7 In practice, most older people will have a mixed picture of incontinence, treat for urge incontinence first then stress.

8 Education: suggest regular toileting and reduce fluid intake to 1.5 L/day, ensure patient is aware of self-help groups where appropriate.

9 Diagnose and treat any urinary tract infections.

10 Referral to continence advisor.

11 Further investigations such as urodynamics, cystometry and cystoscopy may be indicated if simple interventions fail.

Irreversible incontinence

- Pad and pants are the mainstay
- The RADAR National key scheme: the Royal Association maintains adapted toilets across the UK for Disability and Rehabilitation, and they are kept locked. People with disabilities are issued with keys, i.e. RADAR keys
- Conveens for men, good in theory but usually fall off too easily
- Catheters as last resort, to maintain people in their own homes, help carers cope and to protect skin if there is evidence of maceration and to prevent pressure sores
- Support groups for incontinence such as the National Society for Continence website: www.nafc.org

Vaginal bleeding

Bleeding from the genital tract long after the menopause must always be taken seriously, because there may be pre-malignant or malignant disease as well as benign causes. The patient may present with stained underwear or bed sheets. If she is also incontinent of urine or has an anal lesion, the source of the loss may not be immediately obvious; however, the history and physical examination should make this clear. The heavier the bleeding, the more likely the cause is to be malignant.

Ask especially about hormone treatment for cancer or hormone-replacement therapy, which is increasingly common; also trauma (including abuse). Even very old women can be subject to this, either from coitus or from some foreign body in the vagina. Further investigation is the province of the gynaecologist. Causes of bleeding are:

- Atrophic vaginitis, which will respond to topical oestrogen cream.
- Benign tumours, such as cervical or endometrial polyps.
- Trophic ulceration from prolapse or foreign body, e.g. ring pessary.
- Endometrial hyperplasia, which may be pre-malignant.
- Cancer of the genital tract, involving vulva, vagina, cervix or endometrium.

Cancer of the prostate

Prostatic cancer is the third most common cause of death in men aged over 55 years old. It is very common in the over 70s, when it is usually an indolent condition. However, invasive disease has a mean survival time of 4 years. Screening continues to be highly controversial because, despite much anecdotal evidence of improved outcome in individuals, there is no large-scale research data to demonstrate increased survival rates.

Clinical features
- Often asymptomatic.
- There may be lower urinary tract symptoms such as poor stream, post-micturition dribbling, nocturia, but usually only late in the disease.
- If the cancer has spread, there may be back pain or cachexia.
- Rectal examination reveals a hard, craggy prostate.

Investigations
- Measurement of the PSA is readily available, but still lacks sensitivity and specificity.
- The ratio of free to total PSA may give extra specificity. A low ratio implies a greater chance of discovering cancer if the prostate is biopsied.
- Transrectal prostatic biopsy
- Histology following TURP.
- Bone scintigraphy: a sensitive way of detecting bone metastases.

Treatment

1 Treatment can relieve symptoms but does little to prolong survival.

2 Transurethral resection is necessary to relieve bladder-neck obstruction.

3 If there is evidence of spread beyond the gland, hormone therapy is generally indicated, but not all would agree with treatment in the absence of symptoms, even at this stage. Hormonal 'control' fails eventually, possibly due to 'clonal selection' of hormone-independent malignant cells.

4 Radical prostatectomy gives no better results and the morbidity is greater than with hormonal manipulation.

5 Radiotherapy is also used, especially for the anaplastic tumour (even when still confined to the prostate) and for localized metastases.

6 Occasional blood transfusions are helpful for the patient with slowly progressive metastatic disease and severe anaemia.

In advanced disease, the aim is to reduce androgen stimulation of the tumour to levels found in castrated men, with minimal adverse effects. Loss of libido and potency is inevitable; all current approaches are palliative and include:

1 Bilateral subcapsular orchidectomy is simple, cheap, effective, but can have adverse psychological effects.

2 Antiandrogens, e.g. cyproterone acetate 200–300 mg daily in divided doses, now a first-line drug despite the extra cost and risk of severe mental depression. More recently, flutamide has been used, with less risk of depression, but with adverse cardiovascular effects similar to stilboestrol.

3 LH releasing-hormone agonists, e.g. goserelin (monthly subcutaneous injections). More expensive than antiandrogens and must be covered by antiandrogen (cyproterone or flutamide) during the first 1–2 weeks of treatment to reduce risk of 'disease flare'.

Sex in old age

Many people continue to enjoy a sexual rela-tionship until the end of life. However, others stop having sex for a variety of reasons:

• Decline in sex drive.

• Erectile dysfunction, usually neurological in this age group, consider referral to urologist for treatment with sildenafil. However, premature ejaculation less common.

• Longer time to arousal.

• Longer time to orgasm.

• Reduced genital sensitivity.

• Loss of lubrication in women secondary to reduced oestrogen.

• Reduced satisfaction.

• Pain, e.g. from arthritic hips.

• Anxiety about provoking further myocardial or cerebrovascular events. However, the evidence suggests that sex with a familiar partner is unlikely to precipitate a fatal event.

• Disinhibition in one partner secondary to dementia may be off-putting in the other partner.

Advice for patients to maintain a healthy sex life

• 'Use it or lose it'.

• Plenty of exercise to keep physically fit.

• Don't smoke.

• Avoid excess alcohol.

• Use of artificial lubricants.

• Seek help early.

Further information

Badlani, G.H. & Smith, A.D. (eds) (1990) Clinics in Geriatric Medicine — Urologic Care in the Elderly. W.B. Saunders, Philadelphia.

Brocklehurst, J.C. (ed.) (1984) Urology in the Elderly. Churchill Livingstone, Edinburgh.

Bullock, N., Sibley, G. & Whitaker, R. (1995) Essential Urology. Churchill Livingstone, Edinburgh.

Dawson, C. & Whitfield, H. (1997) ABC of Urology. BMJ Books, London.

Dial, L.K. (ed.) (1991) Clinics in Geriatric Medicine — Geriatric Sexuality. W.B. Saunders, Philadelphia.

National Association for Continence website: www.nafc.org

Royal Association for Disability and Rehabilitation website: www.radar.org.uk

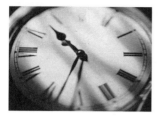

Blood and Bone Marrow

Introduction

Normal elderly people have normal peripheral-blood films. However, abnormalities do increase with increasing age. About one-third of patients will have a reduced haemoglobin. Abnormalities do need to be explored and corrected if possible. Haematological changes in old age are important because:

1 They are common.
2 They aggravate other pathologies/symptoms.
3 They are often correctable.

Age changes

The following facts are given because they are interesting, but they are of more theoretical than practical importance.

Red blood cells

There is evidence of reduced deformability in health and this is even more marked in those with cerebrovascular disease.

White blood cells

1 In elderly people, more marked granulation (probably lysosymes) and lobulation of granulocytes have been described.
2 There is a tendency towards leucopenia, with a normal leucocyte-count range of $3.0–8.5 \times 10^9$/L in old age.

3 The lymph nodes, the lymphoid tissue of the GI tract and the spleen are all much reduced. The thymus is atrophied by middle age but thymic remnants are thought to remain active to extreme old age.
4 The B-cell population is well maintained but there is a reduction in T-cell numbers and functional capacity.
5 Some impairment of phagocytosis by neutrophils and macrophages has been reported.

Plasma proteins

Conflicting reports on age changes relate to the difficulty in distinguishing those changes due solely to age from those due to other factors, such as malnutrition or disease. The main points to emerge are:

1 Low levels of total protein and of the individual fractions are to be regarded as pathological.
2 Increased globulin fractions indicate disease; however, asymptomatic individuals with very high levels of gamma globulins may have monoclonal gammopathy of unknown significance (MGUS) rather than myeloma.
3 Abnormal immunoglobulins are increasingly common in the very old, being present in some 3% of those aged over 70 years and in 20% of those aged over 90.
4 There is an age-related increase in the incidence of autoantibodies and the female preponderance is lost.

Haemopoiesis and ageing

1 There is a gradual loss of active haemopoietic tissue initially in the long bones and later in the flat bones; vertebral marrow persists.

2 The cellular composition of the residual haemopoietic tissue is normal and responds satisfactorily to the usual stimuli, such as erythropoietin, anoxia and blood loss.

Basic investigations

Always request a peripheral-blood film; it is cheap and easy and will often lead you directly to the cause and treatment of the blood disease.

Anaemia is the most common abnormality and the red-cell morphology often suggests the aetiology (Fig. 14.1). White-cell morphology will also be helpful, especially in myeloproliferative disorders.

Measurement of the acute-phase response is also useful. The ESR is the cheapest investigation but it reflects changes slowly (i.e. days). CRP is better for monitoring more rapid changes (i.e. in hours). Measurement of other plasma proteins by electrophoresis is informative when malignant conditions, such as myeloma, are suspected.

Clinical history and examination

The symptoms of anaemia—tiredness, breathlessness and general malaise—are too common and non-specific to be of great value. However, anaemia may exaggerate or exacerbate symptoms due to other pathologies, e.g. angina may become more troublesome, falls occur more frequently. The patient's symptoms may therefore be greater than expected from the documented haematological abnormality.

The history may help in defining the nature or cause of the anaemia. Ask about dietary change, dyspepsia, change in bowel habit, weight loss, family history (pernicious anaemia (PA)), medication and previous surgery, etc.

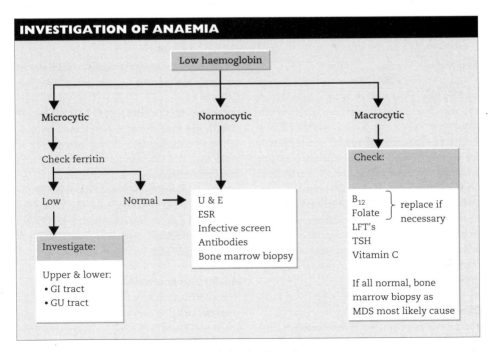

Fig. 14.1 Investigation of anaemia. MDS, myelodysplastic syndrome.

Physical examination may not be helpful but it is important to look for jaundice, lymphadenopathy, abdominal organomegaly, rectal masses and neurological abnormalities, as these may direct you to the correct diagnosis.

Finally, remember that anaemia is a sign of disease and is not a diagnosis.

The types and causes of anaemia

Anaemia is present if the haemoglobin is less than 13 g/dL in males or less than 12 g/dL in females. The main categories are:
1 Red-cell/haemoglobin loss:
   (a) due to bleeding;
   (b) due to destruction (haemolysis).
2 Impaired red-cell/haemoglobin production:
   (a) deficiency states;
   (b) marrow dysfunction;
   (c) anaemia of chronic disease.

Iron-deficiency anaemia (microcytic)

Iron-deficiency anaemia is the most common form of microcytic anaemia. It is usually caused by bleeding, very often from the GI tract.

Aetiology
1 Iron-deficiency anaemia is usually due to chronic blood loss, especially from the GI tract and, less often, from the genitourinary tract or elsewhere.
2 Defective absorption may be a contributory (rarely the sole) factor. Causes include achlorhydria secondary to chronic gastritis, or previous gastrectomy, or small-bowel disease. Look for clinical or biochemical evidence of malabsorption, such as steatorrhoea, osteomalacia, folate and vitamin B deficiencies.
3 Inadequate intake may stem from inability to cope as a result of physical or mental disorder or from poverty.

Clinical picture
The patient may complain of non-specific symptoms such as general malaise, weakness, falls or congestive cardiac failure. The patient may report symptoms of the underlying disease, for example indigestion, melaena or haematuria. The carer may report that the patient is more confused. It is important to ask about past medical history including previous gastrectomy and to document all drug treatments including over-the-counter medications such as aspirin and ibuprofen.

Investigation and treatment
• Peripheral-blood film: the red cells are small and hypochromic. There may also be pencil cells and target cells.
• A low serum ferritin is good evidence of iron deficiency. However it is an acute phase protein and it may be falsely elevated in the context of inflammation in which case the CRP is high also.
• The reticulocyte count can be helpful; if it is raised, this implies bleeding or haemolysis with appropriate increased bone marrow activity.
• If there are no clinical pointers to the source of bleeding, start by investigating the GI tract because it is so commonly implicated. Remember that a benign upper-GI lesion, such as a hiatus hernia, may conceal a more serious lesion lower down, e.g. carcinoma of the colon. Upper-GI bleeding is often iatrogenic, e.g. NSAIDs or aspirin.
• Details of investigation and treatment of anaemia secondary to GI disorders are given in Chapter 11.
• Iron should be continued for 3 months to replenish the iron stores; it is sufficient to prescribe ferrous sulphate 200 mg twice daily, as more than this may not be absorbed and may cause side-effects such as constipation.
• If the response to oral iron treatment is not satisfactory, check that the patient is taking the tablets and that any bleeding has stopped. Also consider additional diagnoses which may explain the problem.

Haemolytic anaemia
A rare form of anaemia in old age and therefore in danger of being overlooked, especially as the peripheral-blood film may not show any specific features, i.e. a variable red-cell size and coloration. In old age, these anaemias are usually

secondary to immune processes, i.e. as part of an autoimmune illness (e.g. systemic lupus erythematosus (SLE)), due to antibody production secondary to infection (hot and cold antibodies following a viral infection) or as an iatrogenic disease (e.g. the haemolytic anaemia secondary to methyldopa treatment).

Patients with hypersplenism may also have a haemolytic element to their anaemia.

Relevant investigations are those indicating increased red-cell destruction, i.e. raised bilirubin level, raised reticulocyte count, haptoglobins and antibody tests (Coombs' test).

Deficiency states causing macrocytosis

The macrocytic anaemias are usually secondary to deficiency of vitamin B_{12}, folic acid or, more rarely, thyroxine. They are much less common than anaemia due to iron deficiency or chronic disease.

Vitamin B_{12} deficiency

PA is the most common cause of vitamin B_{12} deficiency in older people but other causes are gastrectomy, bacterial colonization of intestinal strictures or diverticula and disorders of the terminal ileum, especially Crohn's disease. Strict vegans may also suffer from dietary-induced vitamin B_{12} deficiency.

Pernicious anaemia

PA develops insidiously due to autoimmune gastric atrophy and failure of intrinsic factor secretion. The incidence is said to be 900/100 000 in men over the age of 80 and 2500/100 000 in women over the age of 80 per year. Cancer of the stomach occurs in about 10% of cases. Other complications are peripheral neuropathy, subacute combined degeneration of the spinal cord and confusion, and these may predate the haematological changes.

Clinical features
Clinical features include:
• Symptoms and signs of anaemia, with yellow tinge to skin.
• Glossitis, anorexia and weight loss.

• In severe cases, hepatosplenomegaly, heart failure.

Diagnosis
1 The blood film contains large oval red cells and occasionally hypersegmented neutrophils.
2 The bone marrow is megaloblastic.
3 Serum B_{12} is low.
4 The Schilling's (Dicopac double radioisotope) test will confirm that vitamin B_{12} can be absorbed only when given with intrinsic factor. The test is not necessary in most cases.
5 Antibodies to gastric parietal cells are found in the serum in 90%, to intrinsic factor in 60% and to thyroid in 40% of cases.

Treatment of vitamin B_{12} deficiency
1 Hydroxocobalamin 1 mg intramuscularly every 3–4 days for five doses initially to replenish body stores and thereafter 1 mg every 3 months for life.
2 There is often associated iron deficiency, necessitating oral iron.
3 Blood transfusion is generally not indicated.

Folate deficiency

Folate deficiency is much more common than vitamin B_{12} deficiency and is usually due to poor diet, with or without malabsorption. Other factors are increased demand, e.g. in lymphoma, neoplasm, infection and haemolysis. Anticonvulsant drugs and chronic alcoholism cause low levels by increasing the hepatic metabolism of folate.

Clinical features
The clinical features include:
1 Irritability, depression, confusion and occasionally dementia.
2 Peripheral neuropathy and subacute combined degeneration of the cord (as with PA) in more severe cases.

Diagnosis
• The peripheral-blood and marrow picture is identical to that of vitamin B_{12} deficiency.
• Red-cell folate is low. Folic-acid absorption tests are not used routinely.

Treatment
1 Correct the aberrant lifestyle—poor diet, alcohol abuse; stop offending drugs, when practicable.
2 Oral folic-acid tablets for a few months to replenish stores, then stop; long-term use may mask developing PA.
3 Do not give folic acid until vitamin B_{12} deficiency excluded; otherwise there is a risk of precipitating subacute combined degeneration of the cord. If in doubt, give both vitamins concurrently; the patient may need iron also.
4 Use of folic acid is more hazardous than the other haematinics, especially in the presence of vitamin B_{12} deficiency. May be justified prophylactically in malabsorption states and in epileptics on anticonvulsants.

Hypothyroidism
The macrocytic normoblastic anaemia, which occurs in over 50% of cases in myxoedema, is usually mild, never megaloblastic and responds slowly to thyroxine. Co-existing iron deficiency will require treatment. About 10% of cases also have PA.

Scurvy
The macrocytic normoblastic anaemia of scurvy is commonly associated with other nutritional deficiencies. Vitamin C is necessary for the reduction of folate into its active metabolite. Vascular purpura occurs and on occasion blood loss can be severe. Vitamin C replacement, followed by a proper diet, is curative.

Marrow dysfunction
The peripheral red cells are normally normochromic and normocytic but may on occasion be macrocytic. The underlying fault may be inherent in the marrow itself and examination of the marrow is needed for diagnosis either as an aspirate or a trephine.

Myelodysplastic syndromes
• These are most frequently found in elderly patients.
• Twenty-five per cent are discovered incidentally.

• Eighty per cent present as a refractory anaemias.
• Twenty per cent present with problems secondary to leucopenia or thrombocytopenia.
• The blood film may show a pancytopenia with giant platelets and juvenile neutrophils.
• The marrow is hypercellular, due to stem-cell hyperplasia but poor haemopoiesis.
• A few respond to treatment with pyridoxine, androgens and steroids.
• The majority of cases are best managed with repeated blood transfusions (but remember to consider desferrioxamine to prevent iron overload).
• Chemotherapy often too toxic for use in elderly patients.
• Mean survival from diagnosis is 2 years; the illness may end in conversion to a leukaemic picture or the patient may succumb to infections secondary to poor white-cell function.

Aplastic anaemia
The peripheral-blood picture may be similar to that in the myelodysplastic syndrome but sometimes contains blast cells. The marrow aspirate will show depletion in stem cells. Most cases are idiopathic, but known causes are drugs (anti-inflammatories, antibiotics, thiazide diuretics, cytotoxic drugs, radiotherapy and toxins (benzene)). Treatment is supportive with blood and platelet transfusions, and antibiotics for infection. More aggressive therapies include cyclosporin A, high-dose methyl prednisolone and bone marrow transplantation but these are best reserved for fit people with no co-morbidities.

Leucoerythroblastic anaemia
An anaemia with immature cells in the blood. The marrow examination may reveal the malignant cells that have infiltrated and impaired function.

Anaemia of chronic disease
• This usually a normochromic normocytic anaemia.
• It does not respond to haematinics.
• May be improved by treatment of the underlying condition.

- Seventy-five per cent are associated with malignancy, the remainder are associated with infection or inflammation such as rheumatoid arthritis.
- Ferritin is normal or raised.
- There are increased levels of iron in the reticulo-endothelial system.
- The underlying problem seems to be defective iron transfer to red cell precursors.
- Recent work has shown that anaemia of chronic disease can be differentiated from iron deficiency anaemia by measuring the number of transferrin receptors. They are upregulated in anaemia of chronic disease but normal in iron deficiency anaemia. This is expensive and not yet widely available.

Mixed picture anaemias

Many of these types of anaemia have a mixed picture, with features of deficiencies, blood loss, haemolysis and marrow dysfunction. The blood picture will only improve if the underlying condition can be alleviated. Common examples are as follows.

Rheumatoid arthritis

In addition to 'anaemia of chronic disease', look for blood loss (anti-inflammatory drugs), inadequate nutrition and folate or vitamin B_{12} deficiency. Low folate may be due to reduced intake and increased utilization. Complications of rheumatoid disease, such as vasculitis or amyloidosis, increase the severity and complexity of the anaemia.

Malignant disease

Usually a combination of causes will be operative: anorexia, blood loss, anaemia of chronic disease, malabsorption and haemolysis. Additionally, there may be marrow infiltration, with development of leucoerythroblastic anaemia.

Renal disease

The anaemia in renal disease may be related to the underlying cause, e.g. myeloma, or systemic lupus erythematosus. It is also associated with reduced production of erythropoietin. Elderly patients with chronic renal failure and anaemia are offered subcutaneous recombinant erythropoietin once any iron deficiency is corrected.

Alcohol abuse

Anaemia may be due to a combination of gastric bleeding, duodenal ulceration, dietary deficiency of folate and a direct toxic effect of alcohol on bowel absorption and marrow function.

Myeloproliferative disorders

These malignant conditions are due to uncontrollable proliferation of haemopoietic cells. The predominant cells produced and the speed of progression usually define the nature of the disease. The diagnosis is usually made on the appearance of the peripheral-blood film and marrow examination.

Acute myeloid leukaemia

Very much an illness of the elderly (over 10/100 000 cases per year in the population aged over 75 years; less than 5/100 000 cases per year in all other age groups).

Acute lymphoblastic leukaemia

Mainly a disease of childhood but highest incidence in adults is in the over 75s.

Treatment of acute leukaemias will combine active chemotherapy and supportive measures. Treatment should only be undertaken in conjunction with a clinical haematologist.

Chronic lymphatic leukaemia

This is a disease caused by normal lymphocytes living an abnormally long time. The aetiology is unknown but there is a genetic element; it arises at a younger age in successive generations of some families.

- It accounts for 25% of all haematological malignancies.
- It affects older people; the incidence is 50/100 000 per year in the population aged over 70.

One-third of cases are detected incidentally on a blood film done for, e.g. pre-operative assessment.

This is the commonest of the myeloprolifera-tive disorders. Often a chance finding (high lym-phocyte count on peripheral blood film) and does not require treatment if asymptomatic. Incidence increases with age. May convert to an acute disorder—any intervention should be in conjunction with a haematologist.

Clinical features
- Superficial   symmetrical   cervical lymphadenopathy.
- Anaemia.
- Hepatosplenomegaly.
- Purpura and bruising secondary to low platelet count.
- Often presents as pruritus.
- Occasionally presents as a florid response to Herpes zoster.

Diagnosis
- The blood film contains multiple small lym-phocytes and occasional smear cells.
- There may be a normocytic normochromic anaemia.
- Bone marrow aspirate shows replacement of the normal marrow with lymphocytes.

Treatment
Many elderly people have a benign form of the disease, which requires no treatment, and sur-vive for up to 10 years. The mainstay of treat-ment of those with more aggressive disease is steroids plus alkylating agents. Survival in these cases is usually 3–5 years.

Chronic myeloid leukaemia
Chronic myeloid leukaemia is less common than chronic lymphatic leukaemia. It is of interest because it is the best worked out genetically: the translocation of genes from the long arm of chromosome 9 to chromosome 22 creating the Philadelphia chromosome, which produces an oncoprotein.
- Incidence is 1–1.5/100 000 per year.
- Affects people of all ages, mean range 40–50 years.

Clinical features
- Bone marrow failure.

- Hypermetabolism.
- Splenomegaly, may be massive.
- More rarely, leucostasis causing priapism, and visual impairment; and hyperuricaemia.

Investigations
- Leucocytosis, $50–200 \times 10^9$/L, with the full spectrum of myeloid cells seen in the peripheral blood film.
- Bone   marrow   is   hypercellular   with granulocytes.
- Philadelphia chromosome may be obtained from peripheral blood or bone marrow.
- Normochromic normocytic anaemia.
- Platelet count often raised, but may be normal or low.
- Raised uric acid.

Progression and treatment
Usually the disease remains in the chronic phase for 2–3 years. During this phase, it is possible to treat with chemotherapy and bone marrow transplantation. When the disease enters its acute phase, deterioration may be rapid, with median survival being 3–6 months. It is less common than the lymphatic form but again is found predominantly in elderly population, and splenomegaly may be gross. Again, expert haematological guidance is needed if active treatment is contemplated—usually when con-version to acute form seems imminent.

Other elements of the blood may also prolif-erate to give rise to erythrocytosis and throm-bocytosis. These conditions are rare and their management requires the expertise of a clinical haematologist.

Myeloma
Myeloma is the abnormal monoclonal prolifera-tion of plasma cells in the bone marrow. It ac-counts for 10% of haematological malignancies. It is more common in men than women and in black populations than white. It is a disease of older age, the mean age of onset being 65 years old.

The aetiology is unknown, but possibilities in-clude toxins and the human herpes virus HH8. There may be a genetic component as it occurs in family clusters.

Clinical syndromes
- Malaise secondary to anaemia.
- Bone pain and pathological fractures.
- Recurrent infections secondary to immunoparesis.
- Confusion secondary to hypercalcaemia.
- Renal failure due to deposition of immune complexes.
- Bleeding secondary to abnormal platelet function.
- Rarely: hyperviscosity syndromes, amyloidosis or cord compression..

Investigations
- Normochromic normocytic anaemia.
- Thrombocytopenia.
- Raised ESR and plasma viscosity.
- Hypercalcaemia.
- Abnormal monoclonal plasma-protein band, usually IgG seen on plasma electrophoresis.
- Bence-Jones proteins (free light chains) in the urine.
- Lytic bone lesions on the skeletal survey.

Treatment
This depends on how the patient presents:
- Careful fluid balance for renal failure, and dialysis in selected cases.
- Fluids and bisphosphonates for hypercalcaemia. Some studies are showing that patients treated with bisphosphonates do better in the long term.
- Radiotherapy for bone pain and cord compression.
- It is important to assess the patient carefully before commencing chemotherapy: consider aggressive treatment with a view to bone marrow transplant in younger and fitter patients.
- If chemotherapy is deemed appropriate, the mainstay is melphalan, usually given with prednisolone. Myeloma usually responds to this but then relapses again.

Monoclonal gammopathy of uncertain significance
Sometimes a paraprotein is found in the serum but there is no definite evidence of myeloma; no bone lesions, no Bence-Jones proteins in the urine.

Some of these patients, but not all, will eventually develop full myeloma.

Lymphoma

There are two main types of lymphoma:

1 *Hodgkin's disease.* This mainly affects adolescents and people in their thirties, but there is a second peak affecting 50–80 year olds. Reed–Sternberg cells are pathognomonic of Hodgkin's disease; they are multi-nucleated giant cells found in the peripheral blood. The clinical features include lymphadenopathy which is typically localized and above the diaphragm. It may be accompanied by constitutional symptoms such as fever and weight loss.

2 *Non-Hodgkin's lymphoma.* The incidence increases with increasing age. Any lymphoid tissue may be affected (up to 20% of cases arise in the GI tract, bone, liver or CNS). Symptoms of both varieties are similar—general malaise, pyrexia of unknown origin, night sweats, pruritus and weight loss. Compression of neighbouring structures may also lead to symptoms. Cerebral lymphoma presents with subacute progression of confusion or other neurological symptoms such as dizziness. It is more common in immunosupressed patients.

Investigations
- Lymph node biopsy.
- Blood film: leucocytosis.
- Normochromic normocytic anaemia.
- Bone marrow.
- Raised ESR and LDH.
- CT abdomen, pelvis and chest.

Treatment
Treatment depends on histology and staging. Generally, elderly patients respond poorly to the regimes used and often suffer severe adverse side effects.

Coagulation disorders

Clotting disorders

The clotting problem most familiar in geriatric practice is DVT. Age alone is a risk factor but most patients also have other precipitants, such as immobility, trauma (accidental and surgical), underlying malignant disease and dehydration. Other conditions in which the blood has increased viscosity, e.g. myeloma, polycythaemia, hyperosmolar non-ketotic diabetic coma and hypothermia, are also complicated by the increased risk of venous thrombosis. All patients at increased risk should be offered protection with prophylactic low molecular weight heparin and thrombo-embolic device stockings (TEDS). See Chapter 9 for more information about venous thromboembolism.

Bleeding disorders

The most common cause of prolonged bleeding is medical treatment or overtreatment with anticoagulants. As the indications for anticoagulation of elderly patients increase, so will the episodes of overtreatment. Elderly patients are particularly at risk, because of the problem of compliance (with both drug regime and regular monitoring) experienced by some elderly patients, plus the complication of drug interactions, especially with analgesics, NSAIDs and antibiotics introduced to treat new problems in patients previously well controlled on regular anticoagulants, not forgetting greater risk of falls, etc.

Other elderly patients at risk are those with thrombocytopenia, whether it is part of their underlying pathology, as in aplastic anaemia or autoimmune idiopathic thrombocytopenia, or as a consequence of powerful chemotherapeutic regimes for myeloproliferative and other neoplastic diseases. The risk of serious haemorrhage, e.g. stroke, is much higher in elderly subjects.

The increasing use of thrombolysis, including streptokinase (see Chapter 9) is another example of elderly patients experiencing both greater benefits and greater risks. Careful selection is needed to avoid the increased risk of bleeding, especially cerebral.

Disseminated intravascular coagulation

In disseminated intravascular coagulation (DIC), thrombosis and bleeding combine. The initial thrombotic element is usually silent but the consumption of coagulation factors used in the process leads to uncontrolled bleeding. The likely precipitants in old age are sepsis, disseminated malignant disease, trauma and fulminant liver failure. Only sepsis is likely to respond to active treatment. Other supportive treatments are blood transfusion for bleeding, fresh-frozen plasma for the replacement of coagulation factors and fresh platelet transfusions. In general, 50% of cases die and a higher percentage succumb in very frail elderly patients.

Further information

Bower, M. & Galvani, D.W. (2001) *Haematology and Oncology.* In: *Medical Masterclass* (J.D. Firth, editor-in-chief), Blackwell Science, Oxford.

Hughes-Jones, N.C. & Wickramasinghe, S.N. (1996) *Lecture Notes on Haematology.* Blackwell Science, Oxford.

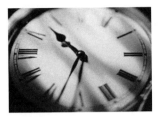

Eyes, Ears and Skin

Eyes

Age changes

1 Eyes appear sunken in old age, due to loss of periorbital fat.

2 Arcus senilis is common but not significant.

3 The pupils tend to be small and slow to react to light, and accommodation becomes impaired. Dilatation is also poor and hinders adaptation to dark.

4 Presbyopia is the deterioration of vision with old age. It occurs because the lens becomes inelastic; so that focusing becomes difficult, particularly on near objects.

5 Entropion (in-turned lashes) is common and causes irritation of the cornea. It can be corrected surgically.

6 Ectropion (out-turned lashes) is common and the most frequent cause of epiphora (watery eye). Again, this can be surgically corrected.

Examination of the retinal fundus in old age

Short-acting eye drops are recommended, e.g. topicamide 0.5%. Reversal with pilocarpine is usually unnecessary and can be painful. The risk of acute closed-angle ('congestive') glaucoma is minimal but beware the small eyeball with a shallow anterior chamber and small-diameter cornea. If in doubt, dilate only one pupil with phenylephrine 10% and reverse with thymoxamine 0.5% and leave the other eye for a subsequent occasion.

Loss of vision

Approximately 70 000 persons over the age of 65 years in the UK are registered as partially sighted, i.e. about 1% of the elderly population (Fig. 15.1). Many more are visually disabled but remain unregistered. Registration of disability is an essential qualification for special supplementary benefits and aids.

Visual impairment

Slow loss
- Open angle glaucoma (chronic), 5%: central vision is maintained until late in the disease
- Cataracts, 33%
- Age-related macular degeneration, 45%: central vision is lost but peripheral vision is maintained
- Iatrogenic disease
- Retinopathy (diabetes mellitus), 17%

Sudden loss
- Central retinal artery occlusion, secondary to embolus from carotid bifurcation or mitral valve
- Venous occlusion: more common in patients with hypertension or hyperviscosity syndromes
- Retinal detachment
- Vitreous haemorrhage, more common in diabetics
- Acute glaucoma
- Ischaemic optic atrophy, secondary to giant cell arteritis or atherosclerosis

NB: If one eye is affected the other is at risk

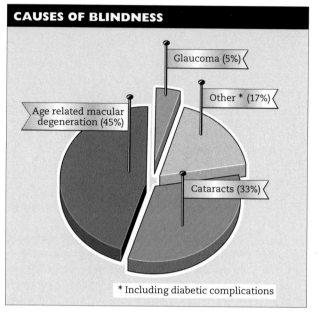

CAUSES OF BLINDNESS

Glaucoma (5%)

Other * (17%)

Age related macular degeneration (45%)

Cataracts (33%)

* Including diabetic complications

Fig. 15.1 Causes of blindness in old age. (*Source: The Challenges of Aging*. ABPI, London, 1991).

DIFFERENCES BETWEEN ACUTE AND CHRONIC GLAUCOMA

	Acute—closed-angle	Chronic—open-angle
Symptoms	Sudden pain in eye, blurred vision, vomiting and prostration	Insidious loss of vision, leading to tunnel vision; family history common
Signs	Eye tense, irregular fixed pupil, cornea and conjunctivae congested	Raised pressure on tonometry, scotoma on field testing; cupped disc
Pathology	Sudden impairment of anterior-chamber drainage—may be precipitated by anticholinergics and mydriatrics	Gradual increase in intraocular pressure—idiopathic
Treatment	Constricted pupil, analgesia, diuretics—urgent action needed	Beta-blockers and/or pilocarpine drops, drainage operation

Table 15.1

The painful eye
1 Closed-angle glaucoma (acute).
2 Infection:
  (a) Conjunctivitis.
  (b) Uveitis.
  (c) Herpes zoster.

3 Trauma, e.g. corneal abrasion or a foreign body.

Chronic glaucoma
See Table 15.1 of differences between acute and chronic glaucoma.

- May result in blindness if not treated.
- Early cases best detected by regular eye tests, with ocular-pressure measurement.
- It usually affects peripheral vision first and only affects central vision late in the disease.
- May affect one eye more than the other.
- The intraocular pressure is reduced usually initially with miotic eye drops, such as pilocarpine, or oral carbonic anhydrase inhibitors, such as acetazolamide, or timolol, a beta-blocker.
- If this fails, a trabeculectomy can be performed with an argon laser or surgically.

Acute glaucoma
- Less common than chronic glaucoma.
- Easier to detect because it presents with painful loss of vision.
- The patient may also describe haloes around lights secondary to corneal oedema.
- Treatment is by laser iridectomy.

Cataracts
Very common, easily detected and corrected, with enormous enhancement of lifestyle.

Types
1 Central—early visual loss.
2 Peripheral—late visual loss and vision impaired by scattering of bright light.

Causes
- ?Ageing.
- Hereditary.
- Diabetes mellitus.
- Iatrogenic, e.g. steroids.
- Environmental—bright excessive sunshine (the reason for increased incidence in the tropics).

Treatment
Surgery
Timing depends on the needs of the individual, e.g. cataract extraction should be done earlier in those who read a lot, but may be delayed in those whom the distortion and change in magnification and reduced visual fields caused by wearing glasses post-operatively would be a hindrance.

Contraindications
1 Early stages.
2 Where vision is compromised by other ocular co-morbidities such as macular degeneration or severe retinopathy.
3 In the presence of severe mental impairment.

Surgical procedures
- Usually done as a day case under local anaesthetic.
- The anterior chamber of the eye is incised. Phacoemulsification is the process of fragmenting the opacified lens by ultrasound. This debris is removed, leaving the lens capsule intact. An artificial lens is inserted into the capsule.
- Ideally, the power of the new lens is selected to optimize vision so that the patient does not have to wear the thick, old-style aphakic spectacles.

Complications of treatment
1 Dilatation of pupil—may precipitate glaucoma.
2 Lens implant—possible failure and risk of infection.
3 Posterior capsular opacification: may occur several months after the cataract extraction and is treated by YAG laser capsulotomy.

Giant cell arteritis
See also Chapter 9.
1 This is a vision-threatening disease.
2 Presents with loss of vision associated with headache, usually localized to the temporal arteries plus scalp tenderness on combing hair, and jaw ache secondary to ischaemia.
3 The patient is often systemically unwell.
4 Examination of the fundus may reveal optic disc oedema with splinter retinal haemorrhages.
5 The diagnosis is supported by a raised ESR

and CRP and confirmed by temporal artery biopsy.

6 The treatment is high-dose oral steroids.

Treatable precipitating/aggravating factors in vascular causes of visual loss

1 Hypertension/hypotension.
2 Diabetes.
3 Polycythaemia.
4 Paraproteinaemia.
5 Arteritis.

Simple measures to assist patients with visual impairment

1 Check visual acuity—provision or change of lenses may help.
2 Keep patient and spectacles together.
3 Keep spectacles clean.
4 Insist on appropriate lighting, a good light is the best visual aid there is. However, some people will benefit from a bright light but glare should be avoided in others.
5 Encourage the patient to be registered as partially sighted or blind. In the UK this is done by a consultant ophthalmologist. The advantages are access to benefits such as attendance allowance, help with telephone costs and cheaper television licences.
6 Seek advice about the availability and use of low-visual aids.
7 Maintain maximum hearing ability.
8 Seek support of blind association, e.g. the Royal Institute for the Blind, website: www.rnib.org.uk.
9 Subscribe to talking newspaper, talking-book library, etc.

Ears

Ageing changes

1 Wax becomes more viscous and needs to be removed in one-quarter of elderly people.
2 Presbyacusis occurs—loss of high-frequency hearing.
3 Recruitment occurs, i.e. difficulty in hearing when background noise exists.

4 Over 70 years of age, 60% of people have impaired hearing and should be considered for provision of a hearing-aid.
5 Impaired hearing leads to impaired health.

Causes of hearing impairment

1 Nerve deafness:
(a) Ageing (presbyacusis).
(b) Ototoxicity—drugs, e.g. gentamicin and frusemide in high dosage.
(c) Nerve compression, e.g. acoustic neuroma and Paget's disease.
2 Conduction deafness:
(a) Impacted wax.
(b) Otosclerosis—hereditary condition, therefore early onset likely.
(c) Post-infective.
(d) Paget's disease of bone.
At present only conductive forms of deafness are amenable to surgical treatment.

Management of hearing impairment

1 Check for wax in ears. This can be removed by first administering softening drops, e.g. olive oil, and then microsuctioning if necessary.
2 If deafness persists after wax removal—refer for audiometry.
3 If appropriate, a hearing aid should be offered (see box below).
4 It is worth asking whether or not the patients think they are deaf. If not they are unlikely to comply with a hearing aid.
5 Inform both the patient and their family about environmental aids, e.g. flashing telephones and door bells, vibrating pillow alarm clocks and smoke alarms, etc. Advise about use of 'T' switch, an aid for use in conjunction with induction loop systems to amplify television, telephones. Cinemas, etc.
6 Educate the patient about national charities and local support groups.

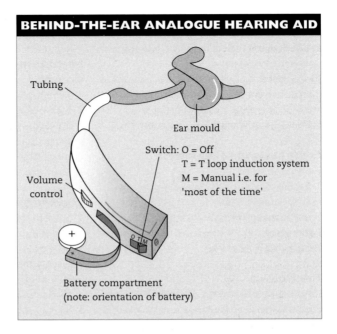

BEHIND-THE-EAR ANALOGUE HEARING AID

Tubing

Ear mould

Switch: O = Off
T = T loop induction system
M = Manual i.e. for
'most of the time'

Volume control

Battery compartment
(note: orientation of battery)

Fig. 15.2

Hearing aids

- It is important to warn the patient that normal hearing will not be restored by a hearing aid at the outset, otherwise people are so off-put by the noises that they do not persevere.
- Generally, people do better the more they practise with the hearing aid early on.
- For people with bilateral hearing impairment, bilateral hearing aids give the best result, if tolerated.
- Ensure ear mould is inserted correctly into ear, otherwise there will be feedback producing the characteristic whistling noise.
- Teach maintenance of aid, i.e. cleaning of tubing and battery replacement (see Fig. 15.2).
- Follow up to ensure that aid is being used — volunteers can help.
- Behind-the-ear analogue hearing aids are the type most frequently used at present.

- Body-worn hearing aids are the strongest available and are therefore still used by people with profound hearing loss.
- In-the-ear aids have the advantage of being discrete but are easily plugged up with wax and are awkward for people with reduced dexterity to fit and they are readily lost, especially in hospitals. They are not useful in patients who have otitis externa (inflammation of the pinna and ear canal).
- The new digital hearing aids have the advantage of being programmed to the individual so that, for example, the frequency of speech can be amplified and background noise reduced. At present, they are not strong enough for people with severe to profound deafness. They are now available on the NHS.

How to communicate with people who have hearing impairment

1 Do not shout, as this just increases the distortion of your voice.

2 Speak clearly and slowly but not in an exaggerated way.

3 Face the patient and make sure that your face is well lit in order to assist lip-reading.

4 Do not obscure or conceal your mouth; to do so makes lip-reading difficult.

5 Ask the patient if they can hear you, adjust

tone of voice or try rephrasing your question, etc. if problem exists.

6 Check that, if patient has an aid, it is properly worn and functioning.

7 All clinics, consultation rooms and wards should have available a simple portable microphone and earpiece, or 'communicator'.

8 If all else fails, write down your questions.

Complications of deafness

1 Social isolation.

2 Psychiatric disorders, especially paranoia.

3 Associated tinnitus.

4 Associated dizziness and unsteadiness.

5 Increased risk of accidents because of reduced auditory warnings.

Tinnitus

1 Noises in ears, may be continuous or intermittent. Often described as a rushing, buzzing or roaring in the ears. If full sentences are heard, then a psychiatric cause should be excluded.

2 Usually due to degenerative changes in middle or inner ear.

3 If the tinnitus is unilateral, an acoustic neuroma should be excluded.

4 Can be noise-induced.

5 Affects over 20% of population over 65 years.

6 Severe symptoms in 5%.

7 Incapacitating in 0.5%.

8 Treatment:

(a) Hearing-aid may help if associated with hearing loss.

(b) Avoid stress and tiredness as these aggravate the symptoms.

(c) Try the effect of a masker, which produces 'white noise'.

(d) Seek support from self-help organization, e.g. Tinnitus Association.

The mouth and its contents

The lips

1 Herpes simplex — as in younger patients, is often an indicator of systemic disease.

2 Angular stomatitis — usually due to escape of saliva due to poor closure, becomes red and sore, especially if complicated by fungal (*Candida*) infection; most common in the edentulous.

Mucous membrane as site of disease

1 Pemphygoid and pemphigus — blisters.

2 Lichen planus — white patches/ulceration.

3 *Candida* — white patches on the tongue or oral mucosa, especially in patients taking oral or inhaled steroids and antibiotics.

4 Aphthous ulcers — as in younger patients.

The tongue

1 Smooth and shiny — iron deficiency.

2 Red and sore — glossitis, e.g. Vitamin B-group deficiency.

3 Geographical/furred tongue — usually of no significance.

4 Fasciculation — motor-neuron disease.

5 Injury — think of epilepsy.

6 Ulceration — think of malignant disease but trauma from teeth most common cause.

The teeth

1 In the UK 65% of people aged 65–74 years have no natural teeth and this rises to 82% over 75 years.

2 Even when surviving teeth and the gums are in very poor condition, attempts should always be made to preserve them. It is important to continue having regular dental review; with age the dental pulp atrophies so caries and decay cause less tooth ache than in younger people.

3 Sixty per cent of patients are unhappy with their dentures, usually complaining of looseness.

4 Twelve per cent with dentures never wear them.

5 The edentulous need to continue to consult dentists — gum ridges recede with age and new dentures will be needed.

6 Dentures should only be supplied to those who are prepared to wear them.

7 Dentures should be left in situ in an cardiac arrest, unless they are obstructing the airway.

8 Dignity and nutrition are best maintained if well-fitting dentures are worn by the edentulous; the presence of surviving teeth helps to secure a dental plate and improves the fit. Increasingly, people are choosing to have titanium periodontal implants to which dental plates and fittings can be securely attached. Unfortunately this is expensive, and has to be funded by the individual.

9 Dentures should be labelled to avoid loss if owner is admitted to an institution.

NB: In wild animals, non-accidental death (i.e. due to 'old age') is most commonly due to starvation secondary to dental loss.

Skin

Age changes

• Confined to the dermis, which becomes thinner, more transparent, more fragile and less elastic.
• The skin in old age is also drier and less greasy, due to reduction in sebaceous excretion.
• There is less subcutaneous fat.
• There is a reduction in epidermal turnover and repair of damage to the skin.
• These two factors reduce the ability of the body to maintain its temperature.
• Reduction in sweating is secondary to both a reduction in the number of sweat glands and in the production by individual glands.
• Reduction in the production of vitamin D.
• Most age changes in the skin are proportional

to the extent of environmental damage from sun and wind or heat, as in erythema ab igne.
• Age-related blemishes of no significance include senile purpura (on hands and forearms), lentigo on the backs of the hands, Campbell de Morgan spots (on the trunk), sebaceous warts (face and back) and telangiectasia (face).

Damage to skin

Leg ulcers and pressure sores are common, serious and expensive conditions in geriatric practice.

Leg ulcers

These are usually situated in the distal third of the lower leg. When associated with varicose veins, eczema and swollen ankles, they are usually secondary to venous insufficiency. When well demarcated and painful, arterial insufficiency is most likely to be responsible. In many cases there will be a contribution from both venous and arterial disease (Table 15.2).

Treatment

1 Keep clean, warm and hydrated. Cleanse with saline, water or chlorhexidine.
2 Debride wound either surgically or with preparations as per local policy.
3 Cover or pack, if large, with paraffin gauze if healing. Use hydrogel, hydrocolloid or alginate dressings if exudate present.

DIFFERENCES BETWEEN ARTERIAL AND VENOUS LEG ULCERS

	Arterial	Venous
History	Usually recent	Often years
Pain	Present	Often absent
Site	Medial or lateral leg or dorsum of foot	Above medial or lateral malleoli
Appearance	Small, clean, punched out	Large, weepy, infected, surrounding pigmentation or eczema
Pulses	Absent or bruits in proximal vessels (not invariable in diabetes)	Present unless obscured by oedema
Proportion	15%	70%

Table 15.2

4 Bandage from toes to knee.

(a) Crêpe bandage in presence of ischaemia or cellulitis.

(b) Where there is a lot of oedema, four-layer bandaging can help heals ulcers. However, peripheral vascular disease must be excluded (by Doppler measurement if necessary) first.

5 Encourage mobility — but at rest elevate foot in venous ulcers.

6 Use antibiotics if there is cellulitis or evidence of sepsis, but avoid topical preparations because of risk of contact dermatitis.

7 Dressings should rarely be changed more frequently than once daily — when healing has started, increase intervals between dressing changes. Hydrocolloid and similar dressings may be left in place for a week.

Cellulitis

This usually presents as painful, red, hot, swelling of the lower limb, and it is often bilateral. If the cellulitis is extensive, the patient may be systemically unwell and have a fever. Care must be taken to exclude a co-existing DVT (see Chapter 5). The most common pathogens are *Streptococcus pyogenes* and *Staphylococcus aureus* but do not forget methycillin-resistant *S. aureus* (MRSA) in cases of hospital acquired infection.

Risk factors include chronic leg oedema, trauma causing a pretibial laceration (remember to check whether the patient has been immunized against tetanus toxoid if an injury was sustained in the garden), and maceration between the toes secondary to Athlete's foot.

Treatment depends on the severity of the infection. If the patient is unwell, then the best management is admission for intravenous antibiotics, usually benzyl penicillin, adding in flucloxacillin if Staphylococcus is suspected. Use erythromycin if the patient is allergic to penicillin. In the case of MRSA, treat with intravenous vancomycin. Oral antibiotics may be used for less severe cases. Treat any co-existing DVT or Athlete's foot as appropriate.

Pressure sores

These are areas of necrosis due to persistent and unrelieved pressure which exceeds the perfusion pressure of the tissues. The affected areas are usually between bony prominences and an unyielding surface upon which the patient is lying. Persistent moisture (e.g. incontinence) and shearing forces (between the patient's skin and the supporting surface) are additional aggravating factors. In debilitated patients, pressure sores may occur within hours but may take months to heal or even prove to be fatal. Prevention is clearly cheaper and more humane than expensive and prolonged treatment. However, in many instances the damage may have occurred before presentation, e.g. during a 'long lie' after a fall at home. If prevention fails, the extent of the damage must be minimized and healing then encouraged.

Preventive measures

1 Avoid falls, if possible.

2 Avoid immobility — in bed or chair; delays on hard trolleys in emergency, X-ray departments, etc. are dangerous.

3 Identify and protect at-risk patients (Waterlow Risk Assessment) (Table 15.3).

4 Relieve pressure when immobility is unavoidable, e.g. by regular turning, mechanical devices (ripple mattress, water-bed, suspension techniques), or protect vulnerable area, e.g. with foam or sheepskin.

5 Monitor the patient's nutrition.

6 Maintain best possible perfusion pressure, i.e. support BP and maintain good hydration.

7 Maintain optimum general health, treat heart failure and maximize haemoglobin level, transfusing the patient if necessary.

8 Keep the skin dry — catheterize if necessary.

Encourage healing

1 Clean the sore, e.g. surgically, by débridement, or chemically, with preparations as directed by local policy.

2 Use appropriate systemic antibiotics if there is cellulitis or evidence of septicaemia; include treatment for anaerobic organisms.

3 Give nutritional supplements, including vitamin C and zinc, and correct anaemia.

4 Do not allow deep sores to become sealed

RISK OF PRESSURE SORES

Build/weight for height		Sex/age		Skin type		Tissue malnutrition		Continence	
Average	0	Male	1	Healthy	0	Smoking	1	Complete or catheterized	0
Above average	1	Female	2	Tissue paper	1	Anaemia	2	Occasionally	1
Obese	2	14–49	1	Dry	1	Peripheral vascular disease	5 5	Catheterized and continent of faeces	2
Below average	3	50–64	2	Oedematous	1	Cardiac failure	5	Doubly	3
		65–74	3	Clammy	1	Terminal cachexia	8		
		75–80	4	Discoloured	2				
		Over 80	5	Broken/spot	3				

Mobility		Appetite		Neurological deficit		Major surgery or trauma		Medications	
Fully mobile	0	Average	0	Diabetes	4	Orthopaedic below waist	5	Steroids/ cytotoxic/ anti-inflammatory	4
Restless/fidgety	1	Poor	1	Paraplegia	4	On table for 2 h	5		
Apathetic	2	NG tube/ fluids only	2	MS	5				
Restricted	3	NBM/ anorexic	3	CVA	6				
Inert/in traction	4								
Chair bound	5								

Add all the score together to determine the risk of pressure sores: 10+, at risk; 15+, high risk; 20+, very high risk. NBM, nil by mouth; MS, multiple sclerosis.

Table 15.3 Pressure sores: the Waterlow Risk Assessment card.

off—pack with non-adherent dressings, e.g. colloid or alginate.

5 If the sore is large, enlisting the help of the plastic surgery team for superficial grafting may be the quickest form of treatment.

Other important skin conditions in geriatric medicine

1 Shingles—the subsequent pain and debility present the most serious aspects of this condition (see Chapter 8).

2 Pemphigus—this is a life-threatening bullous condition which demands treatment with large doses of steroids. Pemphigoid is a similar but less severe condition.

3 Intertrigo—moist seborrhoeic eczema which is often secondarily infected with fungi. It is especially common in obese individuals and where there is close skin-to-skin contact under pendulous breasts and between the buttocks. Improved personal hygiene and treatment with anti-fungal preparations will be required.

4 *Solar keratosis, basal-cell carcinoma and melanoma* — especially in fair-skinned people overexposed to sunlight. See below.

5 *Pruritus* — search for systemic causes, e.g. uraemia, iron deficiency and lymphoma, and infestation; also sensitivity reactions. Unfortunately, many cases remain unexplained (senile pruritus) and can therefore only be treated symptomatically. Keep the skin moist, avoid irritants, and use aqueous cream instead of soap. Mild sedatives may be required.

6 *Drug reactions* — can present as any lesion, from eruptions to purpura. Pathological thinning of the skin secondary to steroid treatment is another common example.

7 *Ulceration* — secondary to trauma complicating other pathology.

Malignant diseases of the skin

Predisposing factor in fair-skinned people is excessive exposure to sunlight.

Basal-cell carcinoma

Basal cell carcinoma (BCC) is the most common skin malignancy. It arises as a pearly papule, usually on the upper face. It slowly, but inexorably, enlarges and if left untreated it becomes locally invasive. Metastatic spread is rare. BCC is easily removed in early stage by local minor surgery but larger lesions may require radiotherapy.

Bowen's disease: intraepidermal epithelioma

These lesions appear as single scaly, erythematous plaques, usually in sun-exposed areas. They are squamous cell carcinomas that have not invaded beyond the epidermis. They are treated with cryotherapy, surgical excision or radiotherapy.

Squamous-cell carcinoma

Squamous cell carcinoma (SCC) is less common that BCC. It presents as a reddened, indurated ulcer, nodule or plaque. SCC often arises in sun-exposed areas, for example in a solar keratosis or patch of Bowen's disease, but also in other situations where the skin has been damaged such as in chronic venous ulcers. It may metasta-

size to lymph glands. Once the diagnosis is confirmed by biopsy it should be excised or treated with radiotherapy.

Malignant melanoma

These are expanding pigmented lesions, again usually, but not always, arising in sun-exposed skin. They require early excision because of risk of metastases.

Hair and nails

Age changes

• *Hair* — becomes thinner and more brittle and loses its natural colour. Baldness may occur in both sexes but with differing distribution. Body hair is lost in the same order as its acquisition. Facial hair increases in women.

• *Nails* — become thicker and harder — onychogryphosis when extreme.

Pathological changes

1 Retention of hair colour is said to indicate hypothyroidism. If the hair is extra dry, this also may a be a sign of hypothyroidism.

2 Exaggerated hair loss may indicate hypopituitarism or Addison's disease, or be a consequence of cytotoxic therapy.

3 Toenails may be neglected because of difficulty with maintenance due to visual impairment, arthritis or stroke disease.

4 Brittle and deformed nails may indicate systemic disease, e.g. deficiencies such as calcium or iron. Clubbing, pitting and white bands may indicate disease elsewhere.

5 Discomfort due to toenail deformity and neglect can seriously impair mobility.

6 Extra care is needed in nail maintenance in patients with peripheral vascular disease and neuropathy, especially diabetics.

Further information

Baum, B.J. (1992) *Clinics in Geriatric Medicine — Oral and Dental Problems in the Elderly.* W.B. Saunders, Philadelphia.

Finlay, A.Y. (ed.) (2000) Dermatology Parts 1 & 2. *Medicine*, Vol 28: 11 and 12 The Medicine Publishing Group Ltd.

Gilchrest, B.A. (ed.) (1989) *Clinics in Geriatric Medicine—Geriatric Dermatology*. W.B. Saunders, Philadelphia.

Royal National Institute for the Blind website: www.rnib.org.uk

Royal National Institute for the Deaf website: www.rnid.org.uk

Willot, J.F. (1991) *Ageing and the Auditory System*. Whurr Publishers, London.

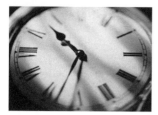

Legal and Ethical Aspects of Medical Care of Elderly People

Introduction

Most elderly patients pose no more ethical or legal problems than other adults. However, in a few, particularly where there is mental as well as physical frailty, problems are numerous. Some of these issues have recently been dragged into the spotlight of the press, with accusations of 'ageism' and 'medical paternalism' being hurled at anyone who dares to suggest that it is sometimes in a patient's best interest to be a little economical with the truth or less than heroic in efforts at resuscitation. Some of the legal aspects are straightforward, some less so, and ethical problems are often very resistant to dogmatic resolution.

Driving in later life

The *law* of the land obliges everyone to surrender their driving licence at the age of 70. A new licence is then issued which is valid for 3 years but which can be renewed every 3 years on completion of a declaration of good health. The *insurance company* may insist on a medical examination. The Driver's Vehicle Licensing Authority (DVLA) must be advised of any change in health status, and certain conditions will render the individual unfit to drive:
• Episodic impairment of consciousness (e.g.

epilepsy, hypotension, severe vertigo, poorly controlled diabetes).
• Paroxysmal cardiac arrhythmia and severe ischaemic heart disease (e.g. angina at the wheel).
• Severe Parkinson's disease.
• Fluctuating or declining cognitive function.
• Uncorrectable visual impairment, particularly significant field defects.
• MI, pacemaker insertion, stroke with good recovery or transient ischaemic attack—for at least a month.

Advice for elderly drivers includes:
• Avoid distractions such as loquacious passengers and the radio.
• If a long journey is unavoidable, make sure of having adequate breaks.
• If the route is unfamiliar, make plenty of advance preparations and allow plenty of time.
• Avoid peak traffic times and night driving.

Ethical difficulties may arise in this connection, and two are particularly common:
1 The patient refuses to accept advice to stop driving in spite of one of the disorders listed above.
2 The patient may have some degree of cognitive impairment but, even though they do not have one of the proscribed conditions, the doctor is convinced they are unsafe.

If the doctor is unable to persuade them to give up driving, a family member may be prepared to try to do so, particularly if they have first-hand experience of a terrifying ride in the passenger seat. Alternatively, the patient may be willing to seek the opinion of a professional driving instructor or, better still, one of the *Driving Assessment Centres*.

Mental competence

The Law Commission has stated that a person is mentally incapable if they are unable by reason of mental disability to make a decision for his or herself on the matter in question, or is unable to communicate their decision on that matter because of unconsciousness or any other reason. A person is able to make a decision if able to understand, retain and believe the relevant information, weigh up the potential risks and benefits, and arrive at a choice, whether a rational one or not.

The assessment of mental capacity is specific to the decision required at the time and should, if possible, be deferred until reversible conditions, which may affect it, have been rectified. A patient is presumed to be mentally capable until the reverse is demonstrated but incompetence will then be presumed until recovery is demonstrated.

Competence and medical treatment

A mentally competent adult is at liberty to refuse treatment for absolutely any reason or for no reason at all. An incompetent patient should be treated 'in their best interests', and the responsibility for deciding what those are is solely the doctor's, and does not rest with the relatives even though it is obvious good practice to consult them. The Law Commission has listed the main factors relevant to determining best interests:

• Past and present wishes, if known, and the factors the patient would take into account were they able to ('substituted judgement'). Very occasionally, these wishes may have been committed to paper in the form of an *advance directive* ('prior autonomy'), which might include the appointment of a surrogate to make such decisions by proxy.

• The need to involve the patient's participation as far as possible.
• The views of 'significant others'.
• Whether an alternative treatment is available which is less restrictive of the patient's autonomy.

Mental competence and research

The recruitment of subjects to research projects is based on identical principles. If the research is therapeutic, the Law Commission applies the 'best interests' test to incompetent persons. Where the research is non-therapeutic but designed to elucidate the basic science of a condition, it is recommended that recruitment of such persons is legal, provided the same information could not be obtained from those capable of consenting, and that it involves minimal risk and invasiveness.

Consent

Consent must be sought for all medical interventions, although this will often be a very informal process and sometimes only implied. Without it, the health care professional has committed the crime of *battery*. Written forms are highly desirable for surgical procedures and research involving drug trials or other interventions, although oral consent is equally valid in law. Consent must be *informed*, which means that the doctor must provide the necessary information, and ambiguities can arise concerning just how much information has been imparted and whether it was couched in appropriate and readily assimilable terms. Consent must also be voluntary, in other words no undue pressure must have been exerted on the patient.

In England and Wales, another person can neither give nor withhold consent on behalf of a mentally incompetent adult, although in Scotland their legal 'tutor' (advocate) may do so.

The role of the court

Where there is doubt concerning the patient's competence, or concerning the best interests of an incompetent patient, particularly where carers and doctors disagree, guidance may be sought from the Court of Appeal. The court does not have the power to issue a consent any more than anybody else but it can issue a declaration that the proposed treatment would be lawful. In considering the patient's best interests, the court will be guided by the *Bolam test*, which simply asks whether the treatment would be supported by a responsible body of medical opinion. An approach to the court is best made through the hospital's legal services manager or, in an emergency, through the duty manager. One source of uncertainty besetting the medical attendant's mind has often been, whether a stated refusal of life-sustaining treatment represents a state of temporary despair which might be reversed after further consideration, or whether it should be acted upon. The judgment in the highly publicized case of 'Miss B' in the UK in 2002 gives a strong steer to the profession that, providing the patient is competent, these stated wishes should be respected however apparently irrational.

Emergency symptomatic treatment of the incompetent patient

In practice, this implies the parenteral sedation of the acutely confused, disturbed patient whose restlessness or aggressive behaviour is a danger to him/herself or, less commonly, to others. As will have been inferred from the foregoing, it is permissible under common law to hold the patient down in order to administer an injection in these circumstances as a last resort and for his or her own protection, if other physicians would regard it as appropriate, and if reasonable people would want the treatment themselves. The procedure is deeply distressing to one and all and can usually be avoided (see also Chapter 4).

Restraints

Sedation is a form of chemical restraint and has been termed a 'pharmacological straitjacket' but may be temporarily necessary in the acutely confused, ambulant patient until investigations

and treatment rectify the condition. With non-ambulant patients, *physical restraints*, such as tying the limbs, should also only be used as a last resort. Patients seldom fall out of bed: they fall while trying to get out of bed, so fitting bedrails ensures that the fall occurs from a greater height than it otherwise would, certainly in the case of confused but reasonably agile patients, and nursing them on a mattress on the floor may be a preferable option. This is not necessarily true of lethargic but frail subjects, who may receive some protection from bedrails, which remind them to ask for help to go to the toilet and thereby prevent them from slithering from the side of the bed to the floor. Tilting chairs should similarly be avoided where possible, but poor staffing levels and a rising tide of complaints and litigation has made the prevention of falls by any means a higher priority for the management than respect for autonomy.

Environmental restraints

Environmental restraints include doors that, although not locked, are difficult to open, or a barricaded kitchen in the home, both occasionally necessary for the individual's protection. A controversial restraint is the *electronic tag*, which triggers an alarm if the patient leaves the hospital ward. This may infringe civil liberties but less so, perhaps, than having your life support systems switched off as you lie in ITU by a disorientated patient who wanders in and wants to plug a toaster into an inconveniently occupied socket. Whatever type of restraint is used, the method, the reasons and the arrangements for review should be documented.

Testamentary capacity and powers of attorney

Testamentary capacity means mental competence in the single connection of drawing up (or revoking) a will. In order to be capable of this act, a person needs to:
• Understand the nature of such an act.
• Have a reasonable grasp of the extent of their assets — so an assessing doctor has to have at least a vague idea of the patient's circumstances.

- Be aware which persons have some claim on their property.
- Be free of delusions which might distort their judgement.

Loss of testamentary capacity prevents the arrangement of a *Power of Attorney*, which enables someone who is competent but perhaps physically handicapped to request a person whom they trust to carry out financial and other transactions for them under their instructions. Theoretically, it invalidates an existing Power of Attorney but, if there is no reason to doubt the good intentions of the attorney, it can simply cause hassle all round to insist on this.

The Court of Protection

A patient who has a moderate estate but who is not of testamentary capacity should have their affairs placed in the hands of the Court of Protection. Application may be made by a relative, the solicitor or the doctor. A medical certificate is required and the Court will usually appoint an interested relative or other suitable person as Receiver, to act as the patient's agent, but not to dispose of assets.

An *Enduring Power of Attorney* enables a person of sound mind to make a proleptic appointment of an attorney who assumes their duties whenever requested by the donor and in any case as and when loss of testamentary capacity has occurred and the document has been registered with the *Public Trust Office*. The donor and at least three relatives must be notified when this occurs, and the Court of Protection may need to appoint a Receiver.

Where the assets only consist of social security benefits, the Department of Social Security can nominate an *appointee* to deploy them for the person's benefit.

The Mental Health Act (1983): National Assistance Act

Section 2 — admission for assessment

- Applicant — nearest relative or approved social workers.
- Signatories — two doctors — one must know the patient (preferably the GP), the other having special experience.
- Duration — 28 days.

Section 3 — admission for treatment

- Signatories — as above.
- Duration — up to 6 months, unless consultant discharges patient sooner.

Section 4 — emergency admission

- Applicant — as above — must have seen patient within past 24 h.
- Signatory — any doctor.
- Duration — 72 h.

Section 5 — holding power

Allows forcible detention of informal patients for up to 6 h by a qualified mental illness nurse if doctor unavailable: consultant or deputy may enforce the detention for 72 h.

Section 7 — guardianship

This is more widespread in Canada and the USA than in the UK. On grounds of mental disorder and in the interests of the patient's welfare, a guardian may be appointed who can cause the patient to reside in a given place, attend for treatment and allow access to a doctor or approved social worker.

- Applicant — as above.
- Signatories — two registered practitioners.
- Guardian — local authority social services or any other person.
- Duration — 14 days.

Section 47 — removal to place of safety

This section applies more to the physically infirm than the mentally disordered, particularly if in danger through self-neglect or if endangering others. The GP may apply to the director of public health for compulsory removal to a geriatric or psychogeriatric ward or to a residential care home. The authority of a magistrate is required and the duration is 3 weeks. The section is intended to enforce removal when it is likely that this will substantially improve the patient's health. It is often initiated by a social worker.

The government has signalled its intention to reform the Mental Health Act in a white paper. The main changes are likely to include:
- Compulsory committal to be ordered by two doctors and a social worker 'or other suitably trained health professional'.
- This to be valid for a maximum of 28 days.
- The provision of a care and treatment plan to form part of the package.
- Compulsory treatment to be enforceable in the community.

Advance directives

Advance directives, sometimes known as 'living wills', present the opportunity to state treatment preferences in the event of future loss of competence, which in practice means the opportunity to *refuse* particular treatments under certain circumstances in advance. An 'unambiguous and informed advance refusal is as valid as a contemporaneous decision'. Although there is no obligation for doctors actively to enquire about the existence of an advance statement, they may be legally liable if they disregard its terms if its existence *is* known about. This poses the obvious practical problem of its availability at the critical moment, as well as the impossibility of encapsulating every possible clinical scenario. Whether or not advance directives come into widespread use, it seems clear that broaching the subject can lead to much clearer discussion of a really important issue.

Ethical issues relating to life-supporting interventions

Cardiopulmonary resuscitation

Cardiopulmonary resuscitation (CPR) is the issue that ferments the most emotion. This is because of massive publicity in the media, which has led to a widespread misconception by the public that the 'do not attempt resuscitation' (DNAR) decision by hospital staff is the major determinant of life or death during the admission. There is a great deal of pressure on staff to introduce this distasteful topic at their first introduction to the patient. Yes, it is important, but it does not apply to death from any disease except cardiorespiratory arrest, and it does not often work outside the coronary care unit (CCU): about 20% of patients survive CPR, but only about 14% will leave hospital, and only 4% of those will be over the age of 75. It is a procedure about which patients, relatives and hospital staff harbour unrealistic expectations.

A DNAR decision should be taken by the most senior doctor available, after discussion with the patient, if applicable, the team, and with the permission of the competent patient, the relatives, regularly reviewed, and recorded in the notes, together with the reason, under the following circumstances:
- Where CPR is not in accord with the sustained wishes of the patient.
- Where successful CPR would be followed by a quantity and quality of life that would be unacceptable to the patient.
- Where the patient already has a poor quality of life that he or she does not wish to have prolonged.
- where effective CPR is unlikely to be successful—e.g. the treatment is *futile*. This would apply to patients with:
  (a) advanced terminal cancer (death expected in days or weeks);
  (b) sepsis;
  (c) pneumonia on admission;
  (d) renal failure;
  (e) hypotension;
  (f) severe disability;
  (g) deteriorating consciousness, e.g. severe stroke;
  (h) arrest due to GI haemorrhage.

However competent the patient, no discussion needs to be held in this situation.

A recent statement on the subject of CPR carries authoritative guidance*. It should be

---

*'Decisions relating to cardiopulmonary resuscitation'. A joint statement from the British Medical Association, the Resuscitation Council (UK) and the Royal College of Nursing, February 2001. See: www.resus.org.uk/pages/dnar

clearly understood that a DNAR decision is not a proxy for other decisions and does not imply 'not for treatment' — the patient will continue to receive appropriate treatment for their condition.

The intensive care unit

The usual reason for considering a request for an ITU bed is to access respiratory support, for instance by ventilation, for life-threatening respiratory failure due to airway obstruction, pneumonia, neurological disorders or drug overdose. The dilemma is to avoid deaths when the cause is reversible (asthma, Guillain–Barré syndrome) but also the prolongation of life when the outlook is hopeless (end stage emphysema, motor-neuron disease). The other considerations are similar to those governing CPR — the patient's and the relatives' wishes, and the previous quality of life. Unlike cardiac arrest, one of the commonest causes of respiratory failure, COPD, is predictable, and will end in respiratory failure, so the patient's wishes can, ideally, be ascertained while they are well. Age per se is not a bar to ventilation.

Invasive methods of nutrition and hydration

The British Medical Association (BMA), supported legally by the historic Bland case, considers that the use of nasogastric (NG) tubes and percutaneous endoscopic gastrostomy (PEG) tubes, and, by analogy, intravenous fluid administration, constitute medical treatment. If unlikely to benefit the patient, there is therefore no obligation to provide it. Where it is not benefiting the patient, it is permissible to discontinue it, although it may be necessary to seek the court's approval, especially in cases of persistent vegetative state (PVS). As in other forms of treatment, the patient's wishes are the key issue and, with incompetent patients, their wishes if known and, if not, their best interests with input from the family and other carers.

No method of feeding is risk-free. Even oral feeding and drinking, which constitute basic care rather than treatment, may lead to choking and aspiration. NG tubes are often associated with reflux and aspiration and PEGs with skin infections and tube blockage — nor do they prevent aspiration. Thirst in the aspirating patient can often be relieved by mouth care. Stroke victims and those with terminal cancer often pose emotive ethical dilemmas in relation to giving or withholding fluids and nutrients. In the former case, except where the prognosis looks hopeless, it should initially be assumed that good recovery is possible and nutrition provided by 72 h after the event in those still unable to feed by mouth. But for those who feel very uncomfortable with a visibly dehydrating terminal patient, it has been stated that: 'The ethical situation is not that the patient is failing to drink and therefore will die but that the patient is dying and therefore does not wish to drink'.

Age discrimination

Ageism is another hot topic, and is said to remain widespread throughout the UK's NHS, despite the measures outlined in the government's National Service Framework for Older People. In a book on geriatric medicine, the easy option would be to make a sweeping condemnation of it as an evil similar to racial or gender discrimination. When based upon blind prejudice, this may be so. But age discrimination is often based on three rational and humane, if misconceived, principles:

• Older people are denied access to high-tech interventions on the basis that they do much less well than younger ones. There are usually studies available that indicate just how beneficial each intervention is for elderly subjects, and to use chronological age as a proxy for cardiorespiratory, functional and cognitive assessment is lazy.

• The potential quantity and quality of life is too low to justify the procedure under consideration. In fact, life expectancies for the otherwise well elderly are surprisingly high, even at advanced ages, and the quality of life of an old person can only be assessed by that person and is consistently underestimated by doctors and others.

• To make such interventions available to older patients is to deny them to younger ones. Not only is it not the role of physicians to compare the moral deserts of their patients but politicians, who are not shy of directing clinicians how to prioritize their waiting lists, should not flinch from accepting the responsibility for rationing when resources are inadequate for all those in need.

Elder abuse

Old age abuse is difficult both to define and to detect. It takes many forms:
• Physical — pushing, punching, slapping, overdosing or withholding medication.
• Psychological — verbal abuse, shouting, swearing, blaming, humiliating.
• Financial — 'asset-stripping'.
• Emotional.
• Neglect — withholding food, drink and warmth.
• Sexual.
• Cultural — e.g. forcing a vegetarian to eat meat.
Studies in the UK and the USA suggest a prevalence of 5–10% among dependent older people.

Risk factors

Victim
• Heavy dependency, communication difficulties
• Behavioural problems, aggression

Shared
• Poor housing
• Poor long-term relationship

Carer
• Excessive alcohol consumption
• Changed lifestyle due to caring role
• Divided loyalties, e.g. elderly parent and child
• Health problems, including psychiatric
• Role reversal — ageing child and aged parent
• Isolation, real or perceived

Although the diagnosis is difficult to substantiate, there are some warning signs:
• Recurrent falls and accidents, unexplained fractures.
• Multiple bruising, especially clear thumbprint bruises to arms sustained while being shaken, or bruises or burns to unusual areas such as flexure surfaces.
• Injury similar in shape to an object.
• Patient tries to hide a part of the body from examination.
• Patient withdrawn, frightened (especially of carer), anxious, makes effort to please.
• Carer complaining of 'nerves' or of being under stress.
• Difficulty gaining access to patient.
• Isolation of patient in one room of home or care setting.
• Refusal by patient and/or carer to accept necessary support services.

Action to be taken
A competent older person has the right to choose to remain in a vulnerable setting and, if they wish to do so, may be very reluctant to admit to what is going on. Any discussion must be held in private and, if there are grounds for suspicion, the matter must be pursued through interdisciplinary channels, as there should be a local lead professional or agency.

Euthanasia

If euthanasia is taken in its literal sense of 'a good death', we must all be in favour, although most are opposed to the practice of the more generally accepted definitions:
• *Voluntary euthanasia*: the deliberate and intentional hastening of death at the request of a seriously ill patient.
• *Involuntary euthanasia*: ending a person's life without seeking their opinion.
• *Non-voluntary euthanasia*: ending a person's life for their benefit, when they cannot possess or express views whether they should live or die.
• *Physician-assisted suicide*: the patient takes a lethal cocktail by him or herself that has been

prescribed or provided by the physician at the patient's request.

All of the above forms of *active euthanasia* remain illegal in the UK, although it is perfectly acceptable morally and legally to administer increasing doses of sedative and analgesic drugs that may, incidentally, shorten life (which they actually seldom do), if the doctor's intention is to provide effective pain relief—the so-called 'double effect'.

To withhold potentially life-prolonging treatment is sometimes called *passive euthanasia* and some ethicists regard it as morally indistinguishable from active euthanasia. But, as we have seen, no doctor is obliged to initiate or continue treatment that they consider futile.

Breaking bad news

There is little evidence as to whether there are right ways to do this unpleasant duty, although there are certainly wrong ones. There are a few generally accepted guidelines:
• A trusted and familiar doctor or nurse (better still, both) should, ideally, do it in the presence of a close family member (unless the patient raises an objection).
• Ensure privacy, identify the relatives and introduce yourself.
• Pre-plan the discussion and sit down to indicate that you have plenty of time. Avoid jargon, do not be afraid of eye contact, physical contact or silence.
• Try not to kill all hope or to give a precise forecast of the duration of the illness. Offer a second opinion, if wanted.
• Do not be afraid to speak of death and dying but avoid forcing the issue and only give as much information as they can cope with, undertaking to meet again.
• Do not strive for too much detachment—patients and relatives often appreciate it if they see that the doctor or nurse is affected emotionally.
• Undertake to continue support and to relieve symptoms.
• Record what was said, and to whom, in the notes.

There is a danger that, in insisting on observing the patient's right to know, we may neglect the patient's right *not* to know. It is usually sensible to take *some* notice of a relative's plea, 'For Heaven's sake don't tell him—it would kill him', but not to be bound by it. But we have all met many patients who make it clear that they do not wish to be burdened with diagnostic and prognostic information, and who firmly answer, 'No, I don't think so, thank you', when we enquire if they have any questions they would like to ask. It is only humane to continue to offer the opportunity but not to force the issue.

There is also the danger that we break the rules of confidentiality by informing relatives without the explicit consent of a competent patient. The team of carers is different, because they are all bound by a similar ethical code, but this may not apply to the manager of a care setting and it is something we should constantly bear in mind.

Death certification

After a death at home the doctor should see the body to confirm and certify death. In hospital, deaths are commonly confirmed by the nursing staff. The certificate is then completed by the hospital doctor, except in those cases where the coroner needs to be informed.

Her Majesty's Coroner

Doctors must exercise their judgement in individual cases but when in doubt ring the coroner's office. The following deaths should normally be reported:
• Death of a person not attended by a doctor during their last illness.
• Death of a person not seen by a doctor either within 14 days before death or after death.
• When the cause of death is unknown.
• Deaths after accidents including falls, misadventure, starvation, severe deprivation (neglect) including hypothermia, poisoning.

• Drugs, whether therapeutic or of addiction, or abuse, including alcohol.

• Anaesthetics, surgical or medical mishap: also when relatives express serious dissatisfaction or allege neglect.

• Deaths within 24 h of emergency admission (unless the GP is happy to sign the death certificate) or within 24 h of an operation.

• Industrial diseases, even if not a cause of death.

• Septicaemia of possible unnatural cause.

• Those with disability pensions from service with the Crown.

• Prisoners and anyone in the custody of the police.

Further information

Anonymous editorial (1993) Do doctors short-change old people? *Lancet* **342**, 1–2.

British Geriatrics Society Compendium.

Emanuel, L. (2002) How living wills can help doctors and patients talk about dying: *British Medical Journal* **320**, 1618–19.

Lennard-Jones, J.E. (1999) Giving or withholding fluids and nutrients: ethical and legal aspects. *Journal of the Royal College of Physicians of London* **33**, 39–45.

Leung, W.-C. (2000) *Law for Doctors*. Blackwell Science, Oxford.

Rai, G.S. (ed.) (1999) *Medical Ethics and the Elderly*. Harwood, Amsterdam.

Saunders, J. (2001) Perspectives on CPR: resuscitation or resurrection? *Clinical Medicine* **1**, 457–60.

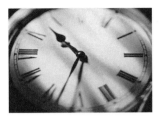

Palliative Care

Age, place and cause of death

Almost 80% of deaths in the UK occur in people aged 65 and above, and almost 65% of women die aged 75 or over. Sadly, perhaps, the majority of all deaths occur in institutions, as Table 17.1 shows.

Ishaemic heart disease, cancer, stroke and respiratory failure are the leading causes of death in the UK and most other developed countries. Of these, terminal cancer and end-stage cardiac, respiratory and renal failure are the conditions which alert the clinician to the inevitability of a fatal outcome, and enable the team to switch the emphasis of treatment from cure to the relief of suffering and the preservation of dignity. Ethical and legal aspects of 'end of life decisions' are considered elsewhere (Chapter 16).

Symptom control

Pain

It is important to try to analyse the source of the pain, as certain types of pain require rather specific measures to relieve them. Examples include:

1 *Neuropathic pain*, in which tricyclic antidepressants, anticonvulsants, such as gabapentin or valproate, ketamine, verapamil or transcutaneous electrical nerve stimulation (TENS) are more likely to be successful than conventional analgesics. Nerve blocks and other specialist interventions may be required.

2 *Bony metastases*. NSAIDs or bisphononates are often helpful. Hormonal treatment usually relieves the pain of prostatic secondaries, and a single bony deposit will respond well to radiotherapy.

3 *Headache due to raised intracranial pressure*. Dexamethasone 16 mg a day is given for a week and then reduced by 2 mg a week to a level of 4–6 mg daily.

4 *Nerve compression*. Dexamethasone 8 mg a day is often helpful, but local infiltration may be considered.

5 *Stretching of liver capsule by metastases*. Prednisolone up to 25 mg a day can be helpful.

6 *Intestinal colic due to bowel obstruction*. Antispasmodics can be used, such as loperamide 2–4 mg four times a day or hyoscine hydrobromide 0.6–2 mg by subcutaneous infusion.

Pain in general falls into the two categories of acute and chronic. The acute type of pain lasts for 2–4 h and analgesia can be given when required in standard doses. Chronic pain, however, requires analgesics to be given in anticipation of the pain and with the aim of a long duration of action; the dose will require titration for the individual patient at that particular stage of his or her illness. In the context of terminal palliative care, it is the latter type of pain which is most frequently encountered. The principles are the same whether the pain is due to malignant disease or to other causes, such as an ischaemic limb which is not amenable to reperfusion surgery and which the patient is unwilling to have amputated. The usual concept is that of the 'analgesic ladder'. This implies a long

PLACE OF DEATH

Percentage of deaths	Location
54	NHS hospitals
13	Private hospitals, nursing homes and residential care homes
4	Hospices
29	Own home or elsewhere (e.g. public places etc.)

Table 17.1

ANTIEMETICS

Name	Dose in 24 h	Routes
Haloperidol	3–15 mg	Oral or subcutaneous
Metoclopramide	30–60 mg	Oral or subcutaneous
Domperidone	30–60 mg	Oral or rectal
Prochlorperazine	15–20 mg	Oral, injection or suppository
Hyoscine butylbromide	600–2400 µg	Oral, subcutaneous or by transdermal patch
Ondansetron	16–32 mg	Oral, intramuscular or intravenous infusion
Cyclizine	50–150 mg	Oral, intramuscular, or intravenous

Table 17.2

and weary climb to the top, whereas in practice the number of steps is usually only two or three:

1 *Paracetamol.*

2 *Failing this, it is usual to use a synthetic opiate analogue.* Co-proxamol (dextropropoxyphene and paracetamol) suits many patients quite well but is very constipating. Meptazinol is often useful and tramadol is relatively free from adverse effects.

3 *Strong analgesics,* which are usually used in a regular dosage regime, often with the addition of less strong analgesics between doses for 'topping-up' purposes for 'breakthrough' pain. In the UK, the principal preparations are morphine and diamorphine, although the latter is illegal in other countries, notably the USA, where hydromorphone is extensively used instead. Diamorphine is claimed to cause less nausea than morphine, and is certainly more soluble, permitting the injection of smaller volumes. In addition to their analgesic properties, these drugs have a valuable euphoriant effect and induce a pleasant state of detachment.

The main problems associated with the use of morphine and diamorphine are as follows:

1 *Drowsiness,* which many patients find highly unacceptable. They can, however, be assured that it usually wears off within a few days.

2 *Constipation* is universal. A strong laxative such as co-danthramer, which combines lubricant and stimulant properties, should routinely be prescribed.

3 *Nausea.* This can usually be overcome by the use of antiemetics, but usually wears off in any case.

Those in widespread use are listed in Table 17.2.

4 *Respiratory depression, cough supression, hypotension* — seldom limiting use of these agents.

5 *Tolerance and addiction.* The former is easily overcome by increasing the dose and the latter can be disregarded as irrelevant.

6 Oral, rectal or transdermal use is to be preferred to *repeated injections* but, if the latter are necessary, for instance due to intractable vomiting, diamorphine is preferable because of its greater solubility and the smaller volumes

which are therefore required. A syringe driver is extremely useful in this situation, with a subcutaneous needle, usually using the anterior chest wall, with the addition of an antiemetic if necessary.

A practical guide to the use of opiates in palliative care is given in Table 17.3.

Anxiety and depression

Minor tranquillizers or antidepressants are used as required, and anti-depressants can also potentiate the effect of analgesics. Psychostimulants (dexamphetamine or methylphenidate) have been found useful in some cases of depression.

Restlessness and confusion

Physical causes should be sought, such as a distended bladder or rectum or a respiratory or urinary-tract infection. If restlessness and agitation persist, a major tranquillizer will be required. Haloperidol 5 mg intramuscularly is often successful and this can be followed by 5–10 mg daily in divided doses.

Nausea, vomiting

It is important to identify the cause: see Table 17.2 for antiemetics.

Anorexia and malaise related to hepatic metastases

Prednisolone 20 mg a day is often extremely successful for these unpleasant symptoms.

Breathlessness

The cause should be identified and appropriate treatment given. The following types of dyspnoea require specific management:

1 *Superior vena cava obstruction.* This is an oncological emergency and should be treated by radiotherapy. Dexamethasone 16 mg a day can be used meanwhile, if there is any delay.

2 *Lymphangitis carcinomatosa.* Dexamethasone is sometimes of value.

3 The '*death-rattle*' due to excretions inadequately cleared by dying patients. By this stage, the patient is generally clouded, but it is the relatives who experience considerable distress as a result of this phenomenon. Hyoscine hydrobromide at a dose of 400 µg 4–8-hourly is injected with the purpose of drying up the secretions.

4 *Pleural effusions.* Occasionally these do not reaccumulate following drainage, but most often they do. It may be necessary to call upon the respiratory physicians to attempt pleurodesis, using, for example, intrapleural tetracycline.

OPIATE USAGE

1 Start with oral morphine sulphate solution or tablets (Sevredol®) 5 mg 4-hourly (if a double dose is given last thing, it should last through the night). Oramorph® solution contains 10 mg/5 mL and there is a concentrated solution containing 20 mg/mL

2 Increase dose until pain relief is adequate

3 Convert to morphine sulphate modified release tablets, capsules or suspension: total dose in 24 h is identical but given in two equal doses. It is common practice to start opiates using MST, Zomorph® or Morcap® at a dose of 10 mg twice a day. MXL has a 24-h duration. A non-opioid or comparable 'rescue' doses of immediate-release morphine can be given for 'breakthrough' pain

4 To convert to morphine injections, use half the oral dose of morphine. To convert to diamorphine injections, use one-third the oral morphine dose (the same applies to intravenous morphine). Usual route is subcutaneous, by syringe driver if needed regularly

5 If rectal route indicated, morphine tampons available for once daily administration using same dose as oral modified-release preparations: oxycodone (Proladone®) suppositories 30 mg 8-hourly are an alternative

6 Fentanyl transdermal patches 25–100 µg/h every 72 h (or occasionally 48 h). Conversion table from oral morphine is available or start at lowest dose: 25 µg/h = 90 mg oral morphine sulphate per day. Permit free mobility

Table 17.3 The use of opiates in palliative care.

Other common causes of dyspnoea, such as bronchospasm, cardiac failure, pulmonary emboli or anaemia, are treated along conventional lines.

Multiple pulmonary metastases, radiation fibrosis and other causes of dyspnoea should be treated using opiates or diazepam and/or oxygen; whichever gives the best symptomatic relief.

Offensive fungating tumours
Radiotherapy is often helpful. The local application of metronidazole ointment should also be considered.

Bowel obstruction
Surgical intervention is clearly inappropriate where there is extensive carcinomatosis, as indicated by liver metastases on ultrasound examination or significant ascites. The 'drip and suck' regime should be avoided where possible in this situation and the pain can be best relieved by continuous subcutaneous diamorphine infusion. Colicky pain should be alleviated by means of subcutaneous hyoscine butylbromide (Buscopan®) 60 mg or so in 24 h. As vomiting is likely to be a problem, strong parenteral antiemetics and octreotide may well be required. A phosphate enema or laxatives can be used to try to relieve the associated constipation, and patients who respond to these measures can be permitted small quantities of food and fluid.

Other problems and some solutions
• *Hiccough*: use metoclopramide or chlorpromazine.
• *Dysphagia*: consider stent or laser treatment for oesophageal carcinoma.
• *Dry or painful mouth* (poor oral hygiene or thrush): good mouth care, treat thrush with fluconazole.
• *Diarrhoea*: treat cause.
• *Constipation*: treat cause, prescribe laxative if using opioids.
• *Cough*: oxygen, opioids, local anaesthetic lozenges, hyoscine.
• *Insomnia*: try to analyse cause.

• *Hypercalcaemia*: treat if symptomatic.
• *Ascites*: drain if causing discomfort.
• *Spinal-cord compression*: radiotherapy if diagnosed early.
• *Lymphoedema*: pressure device, support.
• *Pruritus*: attention to hygiene, use of emollients instead of soap.

Enabling people to die at home

In the majority of cases, it is possible to control symptoms very adequately by means of the foregoing measures. The pain service and the palliative care nurses offer specialist expertise in difficult cases.

In 90% of cases in which dying patients are admitted to hospital (or to a local nursing home provided that the diagnosis has been established and a care plan prepared) the reason is the inadequacy of community support—either because the relatives are unduly stressed or because of unavailability of adequate nursing. Where the community nursing service is unable to meet the increasing care needs of the terminal cancer patient, Marie Curie nurses can augment the amount of support available and advice on symptom control from Macmillan nurses will help to support the primary-care team. Where there is a local hospice, its outreach team can again supplement the care available in the community and may even offer short-term admission for the purpose of achieving symptom control where this has proved difficult in the patient's own home. Practical advice and support are often available through patient support groups.

Bereavement

After the age of 75, 30% of men and 64% of women have been widowed. Four main phases of grief have been described but the stages vary enormously with each individual, and few progress steadily through each stage in a logical way.

1 *Shock and disbelief.* This is characterized by

numbness, disbelief and an inability to accept what has happened.

2 *Yearning.* This phase may be characterized by acute pangs of severe loss and pining and a restless searching for the dead person, who often appears in dreams and hallucinations. Periods of guilt and anger are directed at oneself or the dead person or other family members and friends and hospital staff.

3 *Depression and apathy.* This is a time of hopeless despair, with periods of joyless monotony. It is often associated with profound depression and loss of self-confidence, and guilt and anger are again common features. This emotional turbulence may continue for a year or more.

4 *Acceptance.* This involves the acceptance of the reality that the loved person is dead and that life has changed, and the bereaved person resumes a lifestyle that, to a greater or lesser extent, has become adapted to his or her new status. This phase enables the bereaved person to let go of the dead loved one and to start a new sort of life.

The first of these phases may last for days and the second for weeks. The third phase is likely to last for a number of months, but most people adjust to a major bereavement within 1–2 years. Hallucinations, in which the dead person is vividly seen, may continue for a prolonged period. However, mourning is associated with a number of tasks, which include acceptance of the reality, experiencing the pain, adjusting to the new environment and redirecting energy towards new relationships and activities. An inability to work through the phases of grief is sometimes called a pathological grief reaction and is particularly likely to occur following sudden or untimely deaths. There is a high incidence of ill health and death in the surviving spouse following bereavement. Most areas of the UK now have a branch of the charity CRUSE, which exists to offer help of many different kinds to bereaved people where it is needed.

Further information

Billings, J.A. (2000) Recent advances: palliative care. *British Medical Journal* **321**, 555–8.

Twycross, R.G. (1999) *Introducing Palliative Care*, 3rd edn. Radcliffe Medical Press, Abingdon, Oxfordshire.

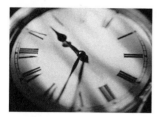

Standards for Long-term Care

Patients in long-term care, in both the public and independent sectors, are amongst the most vulnerable to abuse and neglect. The following checklists and audit systems are recommended.

Patient-orientated facilities and services

Are there separate toilets for men and women?
Are patients taught new skills?
Can patients go to bed when they wish?
Is there a notice-board?
Are there smoking and non-smoking areas?
Does each patient have a lockable cupboard?
Is there a patients' committee?

Privacy

Is it available when required?
Is it available for telephone calls?
Is it available for visiting sessions?

Architectural choice

Is there a shop?
Are there both showers and baths?
Are there chiropody and hairdressing rooms?
Is there a 'television-free' lounge?

Personal amenities

Does each patient have an accessible bedside light?

Does each patient have an accessible electric socket?

Socio-recreational

Is there a garden accessible to patients?
Are there views from the windows?
Is there a visitors' room?

Engagement

Are patients encouraged to maintain skills?
Is self-help encouraged?
Do patients and staff sit and talk together?

Further reading

Counsel and Care (1992) *Not Such Private Places*. Counsel and Care, London.

Denham. M.J. (1991) *Care of the Long-stay Elderly Patient*, 2nd edn. Chapman and Hall, London.

Philp, I., Mawhinney, S. & Mutch, W.J. (1991) Setting standards for the long-term care of the elderly in hospitals. *British Medical Journal* **302**, 1056.

Royal College of Physicians and British Geriatrics Society (1992) *High Quality Long-Term Care for Elderly People*. RCP and BGS, London.

Royal College of Nursing and British Geriatrics Society (1987) *Improving the Care of Elderly People in Hospital*. RCN and BGS, London.

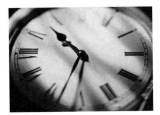

The Barthel Scale

Feeding	2 = independent: reasonable speed 1 = needs help; e.g. cutting, spreading butter 0 = unable
Bathing	1 = independent 0 = dependent
Grooming	1 = face/hair/teeth/shaves all alone 0 = dependent
Dressing	2 = independent; ties shoes; copes with zips, etc. 1 = needs help, but does half in reasonable time 0 = dependent
Bowels	2 = no accidents 1 = occasional accidents/needs help with enemas, etc. 0 = incontinent
Bladder	2 = no accidents; manages catheter alone, if used 1 = occasional accidents, or needs help with catheter 0 = incontinent
Toilet	2 = independent 1 = needs help 0 = unable
Bed/chair transfer	3 = totally independent 2 = minimal help needed—verbal/physical 1 = able to sit, but needs major help 0 = unable—lifted bodily
Ambulation	3 = independent for 50 m—may use aid 2 = 50 m but with help of person—verbal/physical 1 = wheelchair but independent—50 m 0 = immobile
Stairs	2 = independent 1 = needs help—verbal/physical 0 = unable
Total (Max. score = 20)	

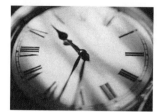

The Abbreviated Mental Test (AMT)

Each question scores one mark

1 Age
2 Time (to nearest hour)
3 Address for recall at end (e.g. 42 West Street)
4 What year is it?
5 Name of institution
6 Recognition of two persons
7 Date of birth (day and month)
8 Year of First World War
9 Name of present monarch
10 Count backwards from 20 to 1

Total (out of 10)

Source: Hodkinson, H.M. (1972) Evaluation of a mental test score for assessment of mental impairment in the elderly. *Age and Ageing* **1**, 233–8.
A score of 6 or below is likely to indicate impaired cognition.

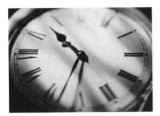

The Mini-Mental State Examination (MMSE)

	Max. score	Actual score
Orientation		
What is the (year) (season) (date) (day) (month)?	5	☐
Where are we: (country) (city) (part of London)	5	☐
Where are we: (number of flat/house) (name of street)?		
Registration		
Name three objects: 1 s to say each		
Then ask the patient to name all three after you have said them		
Give one point for each correct answer		
Then repeat them until he or she learns all three		
Count trials and record	3	☐
TRIALS		
Attention and calculation		
Serial 7s: one point for each correct		
Stop after five answers		
Alternatively spell 'world' backwards	5	☐
Recall		
Ask for the three objects repeated above		
Give one point for each correct	3	☐
Language		
Name a pencil, and watch (two points)		
Repear the following: 'No ifs, ands or buts' (one point)		
Follow a three-stage command: 'Take a paper in your right hand, fold it in half and put it on the floor' (three points)		
Read and obey the following: Close your eyes (one point)		
Write a sentence (one point; must contain a subject, verb and object to score one point)		
Copy a design (one point)	9	☐
	Total score	——

Source: Folstein, M.F., Folstein S.E., McHugh, P.R. (1975) Mini-mental state: a practical method for grading the cognitive state of patients for the clinician. *Journal of Psychiatric Research* **12**, 189–98.

The total score is 30 and a score of 23–25 or below suggests cognitive impairment. A score of 16 or below is suggestive of dementia.

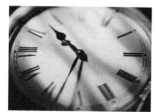

The Geriatric Depression Score (GDS)

The Geriatric Depression Score

Depression is common in the elderly. The 15-point Geriatric Depression Score (GDS) is a useful screening tool.

1	Are you basically satisfied with your life?	No	Yes
2	Have you dropped many of your activities and interests?	Yes	No
3	Do you feel that your life is empty?	Yes	No
4	Do you often get bored?	Yes	No
5	Are you in good spirits most of the time?	No	Yes
6	Are you afraid that something bad is going to happen to you?	Yes	No
7	Do you feel happy most of the time?	No	Yes
8	Do you often feel helpless?	Yes	No
9	Do you prefer to stay at home, rather than going out and doing new things?	Yes	No
10	Do you feel you have more problems with memory than most?	Yes	No
11	Do you think it is wonderful to be alive?	No	Yes
12	Do you feel pretty worthless the way you are now?	Yes	No
13	Do you feel full of energy?	No	Yes
14	Do you feel that your situation is hopeless?	Yes	No
15	Do you think that most people are better off than you are?	Yes	No

Score one point: No to 1, 5, 7, 11, 13: Yes to 2, 3, 4, 6, 8, 9, 10, 12, 14, 15

A score indicating depression includes positive and negative answers but, unless you are very stressed, you will be able to work this out! A patient scoring 0–4 is not depressed, a patient scoring 5–15 requires further assessment.

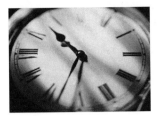

Fitness to fly

1 The partial pressure of oxygen falls at high altitude, even in pressurized aircraft. The resulting 3% reduction in saturation of arterial blood can be significant to patients with severe cardiorespiratory disease, and patients with a haemoglobin level of less than 8.8 g/dL. Supplementary oxygen during flight will compensate.

2 Dehydration may occur because of the reduced humidity at high altitude—fluid intake must therefore be maintained.

3 Extra space may be required by passengers with disabilities: this may be particularly important on economy flights.

4 Patients with mobility problems may not be able to cope (unassisted) with the arrangement of space at airports.

5 Post-operative patients, up to 10 days after abdominal or chest surgery, may run into difficulties because of gas expansion (e.g. in gut or pleural space) at high altitudes.

6 Colostomies may function more frequently than usual during a flight.

7 Epileptic attacks become more likely.

8 Confusion may be precipitated in vulnerable patients by reduced oxygen levels dehydration anxiety and 'jet-lag'.

9 Immobility may precipitate DVT.

Advice to passengers

• Always advise the airline of medical problems so that special arrangements can be made, e.g. extra oxygen, extra space, mobility aids, special diets.

• The cabin crew are *not* nurses—special staff may need to be employed.

• Airlines retain the right to refuse to transport passengers they consider unsuitable.

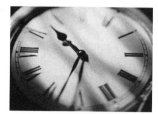

Respiratory Function in the Elderly

FEV₁ AND FVC (MEAN VALUES) IN THE ELDERLY

Age (years)	Sex	FEV_1	FVC
62–70	Male	2.18	3.17
	Female	1.63	2.02
70–79	Male	1.92	2.85
	Female	1.43	1.80
80+	Male	1.97	2.89
	Female	1.01	1.45

Source: Milne, J.S. & Williamson, J. (1972) Respiratory function tests in older people. *Clinical Science* **42**, 371–81.

NB: In the original, values are given for different heights.

FEV_1, forced expiratory volume in 1 s; FVC, forced vital capacity.

PEAK EXPIRATORY FLOW RATE (L/MIN) IN THE ELDERLY (PREDICTED VALUES)

Age (years)	Height 1.50 m (4'11")	1.55 m (5'1")	1.60 m (5'3")	1.65 m (5'5")	1.70 m (5'7")	1.75 m (5'9")	1.80 m (5'11")
65	443	468	483	498	513	528	543
	311	330	349	367	386	405	424
70	435	449	464	478	493	507	522
	301	320	338	357	376	394	413
75	423	438	452	466	480	494	508
	290	309	328	346	365	384	403
80	412	426	440	453	467	481	495
	280	299	317	336	355	373	392
85	410	414	428	441	454	468	481
	269	288	307	325	344	363	382

Source: Cotes, J.E. (1979) *Lung Function*, 4th edn. Blackwell Scientific Publications, Oxford.

Upper figures are for males and lower for females.

Index

Page numbers in *italics* indicate figures, those in **bold** indicate tables. Abbreviations used in this index are shown on page xi of this book.